A COVID Charter, a Better World

A COVID Charter, a Better World

TOBY MILLER

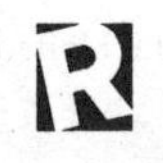

Rutgers University Press
New Brunswick, Camden, and Newark, New Jersey, and London

Library of Congress Cataloging-in-Publication Data

Names: Miller, Toby, 1958– author.
Title: A COVID charter, a better world / Toby Miller.
Description: New Brunswick : Rutgers University Press, [2021] | Includes bibliographical references and index.
Identifiers: LCCN 2020054572 | ISBN 9781978827455 (paperback) | ISBN 9781978827462 (hardcover) | ISBN 9781978827479 (epub) | ISBN 9781978827486 (mobi) | ISBN 9781978827493 (pdf)
Subjects: LCSH: COVID-19 (Disease)—Political aspects. | COVID-19 (Disease)—Social aspects. | COVID-19 (Disease)—Government policy. | Public health—International cooperation.
Classification: LCC RA644.C67 M55 2021 | DDC 362.1962/414—dc23
LC record available at https://lccn.loc.gov/2020054572

A British Cataloging-in-Publication record for this book is available from the British Library.

∞ The paper used in this publication meets the requirements of the American National Standard for Information Sciences—Permanence of Paper for Printed Library Materials, ANSI Z39.48-1992.

www.rutgersuniversitypress.org

Manufactured in the United States of America

Contents

A COVID Charter, a Better World

Introduction
The Year of the Mask

Just as the past is written in its future, so the future is written in its past—aka our present. Just as many historians think of 1848 as the year of revolutions, 2020 was surely the year of the mask.

We stand at an epic moment in world history, akin to the transformations brought about by feudalism, plague, slavery, imperialism, colonialism, revolution, capitalism, socialism, urbanization, war, emancipation, industrialized meat, electricity generation, nationalism, the combustion engine, anesthesia, automation, antibiotics, electronics, nuclear power, decolonization, birth control, human and civil rights, feminism, globalization, and climate change.

We know this conjuncture matters a great deal—it *feels* distinctive—but that doesn't make it easy to understand or to imagine what lies beyond. For COVID-19 "weighs like an alp upon the brain of the living."[1] Only by confronting oligarchic and oligopolistic power, and their extension through deregulation and privatization, can we comprehend and successfully intervene as the conjuncture unfurls, chaotically and frighteningly, before us. The hope is that its contradictions may "'*fuse*' into a *ruptural unity*" and produce real and positive social change.[2] The question is whether those tendencies represent something organic and powerful or something contingent and passing, mere evanescent moments.[3] I suspect they are more than that.

The pandemic is a limit case, an emergency of cosmic proportions that alerts us to the failings of the day, specifically in the elemental field of health. It throws into sharp relief the fault lines of inequality that divide the world both between and within sovereign states, compelling near-universal fear and suffering and raising a vital question: How should we reconstruct our societies, environments, cultures, and economies in the anticipated wake of the pandemic—a world "after" it? To find an answer, we need to examine the dominant discourse of public policy, and health care in particular, then lay out a comprehensive alternative. We need a COVID charter.

In search of such a thing, this wee volume looks at the opportunities, as well as the terrors, that present themselves. It examines corporate, scientific, activist, and governmental actions and perspectives and their impact, notably on disadvantaged, vulnerable communities, drawing on particular cases as well as the wider (im)balance of geopolitical power to consider how we got here, what is going on, and what might come next. Then it looks at various manifestos and charters to help form a new set of rights that could emerge from this otherwise sorry story.

The cases come from two wealthy countries (the United States and Britain) that were supposedly well prepared for such a pandemic but were devastated by it and two poorer nations (Mexico and Colombia) from the region that has been most affected. As of mid-January 2021, the Americas accounted for over half the world's new infections and 45 percent of fatalities. This from nations that make up a tenth of the global population. Mexican deaths were up 19 percent in the previous week, and the United States was up by 20 percent.

Colombia reported a 26 percent increase in contagion. With over four hundred thousand new infections and an uptick of 51 percent in fatalities, the United Kingdom fell behind only its craven gringo partner in the Anglo world.[4]

I have lived in these four places over the past three decades, serially experiencing excellent private health care in New York and LA, thanks to my employment; good public care in London, courtesy of my citizenship; and no work insurance or access to socialized medicine in Cartagena de Indias and Mexico City, as a consequence of being a damn foreigner.

Moving across the conceptual and geographical board, the chapters to come deploy the human sciences as grids of investigation, alongside a few personal stories. The agenda and mode of analysis derive from epidemiology, public health, political economy, sociology, literature, area studies, political theory, science, anthropology, environmental studies, philosophy, and history. I commingle these disciplines under the sign of a materialist analysis committed to progressive change.

That involves looking at structural determinations on people vis-à-vis/versus their agency and transformations in the natural world. As Marx put it, "Man [*sic*] makes his own history, but he does not make it out of the whole cloth; he does not make it out of conditions chosen by himself."[5] Dominant forces secure consent to the political-economic order through a hegemony that makes prevailing social relations appear inevitable, with new norms propagated by emergent classes or co-opted by elites.[6]

That said, material manifestations of power do not simply accrete bourgeois dominance or state authority—consider life in schools, prisons, allotments, libraries, cafés, hospitals, laboratories, arenas, changing rooms, waste dumps, music festivals, mass transit, art galleries, beaches, leather bars, dormitories, railway sidings, dating sites, newsrooms, or asylums. They may be shaped by such power but also deviate from it quite radically.[7]

And hundreds of millions of people live and work in the Global South's informal sector. Immensely underprivileged but economically very active, they neither contribute to taxation nor benefit from it. Rarely the targets or recipients of public policies, these workers ply their trade outside the purportedly prevailing norms of housing, nutrition, health care, savings, and education. That leaves them particularly vulnerable at times of crisis.[8] Ironically, similar problems affect people laboring in the *most* formal sector of the economy—prisons. Although dominated by governments in their economic activity, they suffer in similar ways to the informal proletariat.[9] Or consider the situation of women. Across history and geography, they have experienced pandemics as moments of increased caregiving, heightened male violence, and diminished economic security and decision-making.[10]

The problem with many logics applied to COVID-19 is their failure to address these huge populations as starting points. Instead, they are subsumed by the imagined middle-class rational calculator so beloved of neoliberalism and taken as its purported fons et origo. So as background, I sought to understand the pandemic experiences of workers, prisoners, refugees, women, racial and sexual minorities, children, migrants, the disabled, medical staff, and slave descendants—what they share and what is unique to them and their surroundings.[11]

Beyond that, in order to comprehend COVID, we need to see that the natural and social worlds are irredeemably intertwined. Engels recognized that "nature does not just exist"; it "*comes into being* and passes *away*."[12] He noted anthropocentrism's peculiar faith in "the *absolute immutability of nature*;"[13] hence Adorno ambivalently defining the

Enlightenment as "the progressive technical domination of nature."[14] Those words signify the putative need and right to manage or eradicate vulnerability to harsh climates and food shortages—and to shape polities. From plutocracy to patriarchy, appeals to channel or protect nature—to govern it—are crucial. Bruno Latour avows that "every type of politics has been defined by its relation to nature, whose every feature, property, and function depends on the polemical will to limit, reform, establish, short-circuit, or enlighten public life."[15] As a consequence, theorists should allocate equal and overlapping significance to environmental, social, and intellectual forces;[16] Latour regards COVID as "a global catastrophe that has come . . . from within."[17]

Back to 1848. In addition to revolutions, it was also a year of typhus: a terrible epidemic devastated Upper Silesia. Rudolf Virchow, the founding figure of social medicine who was an attending physician there, wrote a famous report detailing the litany of administrative failures that had mismanaged the crisis. He memorably insisted that "politics is medicine writ large."[18] Getting on for two centuries later, we can see how right Virchow was—that the key element of COVID-19 is "making live and letting die."[19]

The latest, and most germane, form of the social medicine he pioneered is syndemics. It emerged in the 1990s to examine the complex interaction of sequential disease and comorbidity, social inequality, and the physical environment.[20] The *Lancet* proposes that responses to the 2020 crisis "focused on cutting lines of viral transmission, thereby controlling the spread of the pathogen." That's understandable. But "the story of COVID-19 is not so simple": "Two categories of disease are interacting within specific populations—infection with severe acute respiratory syndrome coronavirus 2 . . . and an array of non-communicable diseases . . . clustering within social groups according to patterns of inequality deeply embedded in our societies. The aggregation of these diseases on a background of social and economic disparity exacerbates the adverse effects of each separate disease. COVID-19 is not a pandemic. It is a syndemic."[21]

Syndemic analysis reminds us that we confront an even more horrifying, if slower-moving, environmental specter—an apocalyptic vision that one day there may be nothing left, nothing else, nothing beyond; what Kant called "the shadows of the boundless void."[22] This syndemic was not directly caused by climate change, but its propulsion around the world was produced by the same forces that wreak environmental havoc. For COVID-19 is both a natural artifact and an "unintended consequence" of human action.[23] It relies not merely on evolution but on various entirely unnecessary social relations, such as the industrialized miscultivation, slaughter, distribution, and consumption of our fellow animals, alongside and as part of globalization, culture, capitalism, nationalism, carnivorism, masculinity, and government.[24] The reality of ecological peril is made shudderingly shocking by the COVID alarm clock / mnemonic: even the oleaginous, self-anointed World Economic Forum admits that the inequality both indexed and created by the virus renders our climate crisis more complex to comprehend and counter.[25]

The syndemic's rapid spread and deep impact have been wider-ranging and more sudden than any event in our collective lifetimes, from new working norms to everyday fears about citizen interactions that were formerly taken for granted.[26] In Arundhati Roy's words, "Who can think of kissing a stranger, jumping on to a bus or sending their child to school without feeling real fear? Who can think of ordinary pleasure and not assess its risk?"[27] This pulverizing syndemic is instant and directly threatening, but for all its tragedy, the crisis provides the opportunity to remake ourselves and our future, courtesy of a conjuncture generated by forces of nature and exchange.

Careful reflection on quotidian actions and their links to health encourages a longer view of the life of material objects and the social relations that connect them to us—how the human world transforms, transports, and transmits nature. Our best exit from this crisis will necessitate working with, rather than against, the environment and heading toward a "new social establishment" minus the "antediluvian giants" of capital.[28]

Of course, we should not protect a coronavirus eo ipso because it is part of the natural world. Amartya Sen favors a midpoint between that ecocentric view and anthropocentrism: "The impact of the environment on human lives must be among the principal considerations in assessing the value of the environment. To take an extreme example, in understanding why the eradication of smallpox is not viewed as an impoverishment of nature (we do not tend to lament: 'the environment is poorer since the smallpox virus has disappeared')."[29] One might protect sharks' lives while recognizing the occasional devastation they cause to a tiny number of humans, but a virus that destroys the very life it inhabits is something else. At the same time, the knowledge that emerges from trying to understand a deadly disease can have application beyond the immediate issue of surviving it, in terms of medical treatment and political transformation.

This is especially true of the environment. Consider the tragic cull of mink in Spain, the Netherlands, and Denmark, necessary at an obvious level because COVID-19 evolved toward zoonotic transmission from them to us in a way that threatened treatments and vaccines—the mink variant, C5, was robustly resistant to antibodies created to counter it.[30] But at a more profound level, this was necessary because of the wholesale husbandry and slaughter of the mink, undertaken to suit the fashion industry in farms that institutionalize breathtaking brutality. In the United States, thousands have been left to die agonizing deaths from the virus.[31] And mink escaping these savage culls have the potential to infect other creatures living in the wild or domesticated animals, thereby generating a permanent reservoir of variants with the capacity to transfer to humans.[32]

The current syndemic is just the latest in a long line of diseases imperiling human life as a consequence of meat and fashion capitalism's industrial ways.[33] Of the fifteen hundred known human pathogens, two-thirds are zoonotic. Eighty billion animals are slaughtered for food and clothing every year. They are "Petri dishes for the viruses and bacteria that evolve into a lethal human pathogen every decade or so. This year the bill came due and it was astronomical."[34] Even the International Livestock Research Institute recognizes that zoonotic transmission is heightened by unsustainable demands for meat, intensive farming, and animal exploitation combined with climate change.[35] And when viruses are forged from RNA rather than DNA, as is COVID-19, they can evolve rapidly.[36]

Nature's duality—that it is self-generating and sustaining, yet its continuation is contingent on human rhetoric and despoliation—makes both sides vulnerable. Without nature, there can be no humanity, while changes in the material world caused by people and their tools compromise the survival of the planet's most skillful and willful, productive and destructive, inhabitant. This terrifying time, this year of the mask, may yet prove providential for the environment, if we learn the lesson that human economic priorities have helped produce the disaster, not just evolution. But so far, governmental programs designed to ameliorate the syndemic have "overwhelmingly supported the status quo or fostered new high-carbon investments."[37] Oil prices initially plummeted because of lockdowns, but many natural resources remained in demand, and carbon emissions rose sharply in the second half of 2020.[38] The construction of putatively green infrastructure as part of a recovery from the virus will require massive use of fossil fuels through employment and travel. Goldman Sachs gleefully proclaims COVID-19 "a structural catalyst for a commodity supercycle."[39]

On November 9, 2020—the anniversary of the Berlin Wall breached, *Rolling Stone* magazine's first edition, the horror of *Kristallnacht*, the birth of Spiro Agnew, and the deaths of Neville Chamberlain and Charles de Gaulle—Pfizer and BioNTech modestly declared "a great day for science and humanity": their promulgation of a potentially safe and effective vaccine against COVID-19 that had passed rigorous clinical trials.[40] "We" were a "significant step closer to providing people around the world with a much-needed breakthrough to help bring an end to this global health crisis."[41] *Forbes Mexico* highlighted stock-market advances for the firms involved and other capitalist interests.[42] Morgan Stanley suggested global sales would reach $13 billion.[43] Pfizer's head made millions by immediately selling three-quarters of his stock.[44]

The *Economist* welcomed the vaccine breakthrough as a "shot that rang across the world," troping the start of the Revolutionary War, and "the beginning of the end,"[45] per Churchill calling 1942 "not the end . . . not even the beginning of the end, but . . . perhaps the end of the beginning," to nervous titters from his parliamentary audience.[46]

Director of the National Institute of Allergy and Infectious Diseases Anthony Fauci told adoring Brooklynites, who had just declared him "a COVID-19 hero," "We're going to get over this together."[47] BioNTech's head advised that the virus would not survive the vaccine because T cells will "bash it over the head and eliminate it."[48] News of a second viable drug emerged a week later.[49] The "global race for a vaccine" had sixty candidates vying for primacy.[50] Folk knowledge claiming mass allergic reactions to the vaccines was rapidly disproven, at least provisionally, although some disturbing cases fueled anxiety and skepticism.[51] We were told of clinical trials underway into the antibody therapy AZD7442 that could grant immediate immunity and be used as an emergency treatment to minimize contagion among populations exposed to infection at home, in college campuses, in prisons, or at work.[52] Tedros Adhanom Ghebreyesus, the WHO's director general, discerned "rays of light" and "an opportunity to beat history."[53] The 2021 Papal New Year blessing saw Jorge Mario Bergoglio announce a "year of hope."[54]

Is it "the beginning of the end"? Are we "going to get over this together"? And who is this "we"?

Within just moments of Pfizer-BioNTech's announcement, the new protoproduct had been ordered en masse by the Global North—without prior evaluation in scholarly journals. The firms anticipated manufacturing 1.3 billion doses in 2021—and 1.1 billion of them were secured in advance by Japan, the European Union (EU), Canada, and the United States. Because the first vaccine had to be stored at −70° Celsius, only ultracold freezers would suffice—a further problem for the Global South, mitigated by the emergence of more robust vaccines, from Sputnik V to Moderna. Some alternatives boasted research that validated their efficacy and safety, while others expected us to trust in press releases.[55]

The Gavi COVAX Advance Market Commitment undertook to share vaccines and inoculate the poorest fifth of the world's population through an aid program funded by the wealthiest. But the People's Vaccine Alliance, composed of Frontline AIDS, Global Justice Now, OXFAM, and Amnesty International, warned about the ongoing impact of hoarding by rich nations. Canada's government had already secured access to hundreds of millions of doses for its thirty-eight million people.[56] The People's Vaccine Alliance estimated that seventy countries in the Global South would inoculate fewer than 10 percent of their populations in 2021, because the Global North buying most of the supplies for its own use militated against COVAX meeting its commitments before 2022. COVAX members took a somewhat more sanguine view.[57] Meanwhile, the environmental impact of hydrofluorocarbon gases, freezers, vehicles, and airplanes storing and transporting vaccines and hundreds of millions of syringes and vials turning into waste was daunting.[58]

As wealthy governments scrambled to vaccinate, there was uncertainty as to whether they could viably reduce ideal doses and change the schedules adopted in clinical trials in order to protect as many people as possible as quickly as possible.[59] Within weeks of describing "rays of light," Adhanom Ghebreyesus accused big pharma of privileging places "where the profits are highest," signing dozens of bilateral deals, sending the price of inoculation up, and creating "another brick in the wall of inequality between the world's haves and have-nots."[60] In early 2021, the WHO's Independent Panel for Pandemic Preparedness and Response expressed "grave concern at the prospect of inequitable vaccine rollout around the world." Inoculating a small percentage of the world's population would be neither just nor effective as a means of controlling the syndemic.[61] The world was "on the brink of a catastrophic moral failure."[62]

Word spread of D614G, a change in the genetic structure of COVID-19's spike protein that rapidly became the dominant form of the virus. It was followed by other transformations. Such mutations are to be expected—they are the reason for annual revisions to vaccines against influenza—and may even eventually render viruses less perilous. But this instance increased the spread of infection across populations with astounding rapidity, possibly even among children previously deemed relatively safe from the virus's effects. Reassurances were quickly given that it would be no more destructive than the first strain—that the vaccines produced for the original COVID-19 would probably prove effective against the new substitution and the innovative RNA base to some inoculations could readily be transformed to account for mutations.[63] Then came a revised view: the new mutations might be deadlier than their ancestors.[64]

The sense of an indestructible organism taking over the globe merged with incomplete knowledge, incompetence, and unfairness in the allocation of vaccines and conflictual quarantine and lockdown policies, adding to the despair. Delays in manufacturing and supply, the proliferation of misinformation, diverse regulatory processes, plutocratic norms, and the increased severity of the crisis all worked against the technical efficacy of vaccines translating into real and rapid relief.

All these problems derive from a mixture of untrammeled capitalism and underresourced governments—the product of five decades of neoliberal misrule. For this to be truly "the beginning of the end," we must recognize the crisis of COVID-19 as an indictment of neoliberalism's hegemonic status in politics, international organizations, academia, think tanks, and the bourgeois media. We must acknowledge the profound global inequality over which it has presided.

The argument to come calls for an end to that socially bankrupt form of reasoning, specifically market-based health care. It argues for a reallocation of resources away from pharmaceutical corporations and insurance companies and toward welfare as a universal right. My hope is that the current conjuncture may even dispatch neoliberalism to its deserved home in the dustbin of history—with no option to recycle. Then this might well be, indeed, the beginning of the end.

1
Before the Crisis

In October 2019, the geniuses over at the Global Health Security Index (based in the United States and the United Kingdom, most notably Johns Hopkins and the *Economist*) notoriously declared their countries to be the best prepared in the world to deal with a pandemic. Britain soared with the highest-flying birds in its capacity for "RAPID RESPONSE AND MITIGATION," while the United States was—hold your breath—ranked first for its "SUFFICIENT AND ROBUST HEALTH SYSTEM TO TREAT THE SICK."[1] Mexico was rated twenty-eighth in the world overall, Colombia sixty-fifth.[2]

In January 2021, the United States unquestionably led the world, with 24.5 million confirmed COVID cases and 400,000 deaths; a rich country that boasted a quarter of the world's cases, a fifth of the world's deaths—and 4 percent of the world's population. Why? Why did Britain have more than three and a half million cases and ninety-six thousand dead? And why were Colombia and Mexico also in the top twelve, with three and a half million cases between them?[3] How come the Index was so wrong? Microbes aside, how did we get to where we are?

The picture certainly didn't have to be that way. *Pace* the horrors of war and imperialism, the last four hundred years have expanded governmental protections of their populations from what Thomas Hobbes described as "continual fear and danger of violent death," a "solitary, poor, nasty, brutish, and short" life.[4] That changed across the eighteenth and nineteenth centuries because productivity and health were linked to environment and geography via state and scholarly research, measurements, estimates, forecasts, and plans.[5]

Controlling territory became a secondary priority for European governments, behind understanding and controlling material things and social relations. People displaced princes as sites for accumulating power under the sign of "the economy," an anthropomorphized place of social intervention and achievement that could be comprehended statistically. Cities, countries, and empires substituted for households, with all the hierarchical dislocation that implies. The tasks of government were increasingly conceived and actualized in terms of climate, disease, education, industry, finance, custom, war, and disaster—literally, a concern with life and death and what could be calculated and managed between them. Wealth and health became goals to be attained through the disposition of capacities across the population, and "biological existence was reflected in political existence." The "imperative of health" was "the duty of each and the objective of all." Managing bodies was critical to running countries and empires, with "the life of the species . . . wagered on its own political strategies." This biopower brought "life and its mechanisms into the realm of explicit calculations," making "knowledge-power an agent of transformation of human life."[6]

An emergent capitalism was articulated to the modern state's desire to deliver a docile and healthy labor force to business—but not only to business, and not merely in a way that showed the lineage of that desire. Cholera, sanitation, and prostitution were figured as problems for governments to address through "the emergence of the health and physical well-being of the population in general as one of the essential objectives of political power."[7] The entire "social body" was assayed and treated in the name of "efficiency."[8] So even as revolutionary France was embarking on a regime of slaughter, public-health campaigns were also underway.[9] And while the U.K. Parliament considered the Reform Bill of 1832 that definitively denied the vote to women, thirty thousand of its citizens were dying from cholera. Brought back from imperial outposts, the disease raced through factories assigned to manufacture goods from plundered resources. As doctors tried to explain what was happening, where, and to whom, they began what became epidemiology and interventions associated with it.[10] In 1853, the British Parliament enacted legislation requiring smallpox vaccinations for children, a landmark in the uptake of medical knowledge and regulation of the body politic—and antivaccine protests.[11]

Karl Polanyi referred to a "discovery of society" in the nineteenth century as the moment when paupers came to be marked as part of the social world and hence deserving of attention and aid.[12] Collective well-being was progressively incorporated into European national identity via rights, problems, statistics, and laws. Science and government combined in new environmental-legal relations under the sign of civic management and economic productivity. Achille Guillard invented "demography" in the 1850s, merging "political arithmetic" with "political and natural observations."[13] The new knowledge codified reproduction, aging, migration, public health, and ecology. Biopower gave Europe new life while it colonized and pauperized Asia and Africa.

Over the next eighty years, "Western" society was held to be simultaneously the incarnation of the market and its transcendence. Along came public education, mothers' pensions, and U.S. Civil War widows' benefits—and with the Great Depression, some level of social security. The crisis of the 1930s and the diffusion of Keynesianism ushered "the economy" into popular knowledge as an entity with needs and feelings.[14] From that time, "it" began to thrive and suffer in bodily and emotional ways as if it were a person and hence subject to biopolitical evaluation and intervention. Press attention shifted from relations between producers and consumers of goods onto relations between different material products of labor—a change in emphasis from use value to exchange value.[15]

During the Second World War, with the Depression still wreaking havoc on everyday life, industrialized democratic states of the Global North effectively said to young proletarian men, "We are asking you to get yourselves killed, but we promise you that when you have done this, you will keep your jobs until the end of your lives."[16] That guarantee was kept for decades. Keynesian reconstruction from 1945 to 1973 developed the welfare state across Western Europe and the United States alongside expanded unions, wages, higher education, and civil rights, albeit on an unequal basis in terms of place and social identity. Wealth was redistributed downward, and governments maintained demand and manipulated interest rates to keep economies buoyant.

My parents were born just after the spread of the Kansas Flu, aka the "Spanish Influenza." It claimed more lives than the number of soldiers killed in the two World Wars. One hundred million perished, and life expectancy in the United States dropped by twelve years.[17] Children of the Depression and World War II, my mother and father grew up in poverty, then lost countless loved ones of their generation to battles waged in other countries. By the time all that was over, they, and hundreds of millions of others, wanted a better life for themselves and everyone else who had been on the right side of history. That happened for many of them. My father got an education, and by the time I was born, toward the end of the baby boom, we were middle class. It's a typical but far from universal White working-class story of the time—a tale of upward mobility and an appreciation of the need to care for those without that gift. Full employment was a mantra.

The 1960s saw a rich proliferation of radical protest emerging from new social movements. They were founded on relative affluence, an embrace of difference and equality, an unpopular war, Pan-African resistance, second-wave feminism, and the suddenly international and instantaneous demotic spread of freedom symbols through television, film, radio, and music, from El Che's beret to *Easy Rider*'s motorbikes. Britain withdrew from East of Suez; looked as though it might recognize that its tyranny had faded and failed, as per the disasters of Suez, Kenya, Malaya, and Cyprus; and decided to join Europe. The U.S. war in Vietnam was opposed by millions of its citizens, and a "Great Society" was promised. Third World revolution was in the air. The 1970s were set to be the moment when the Global North's spirited rebellions of the previous decade might find fulfillment along with the Global South's struggles for independence.

Instead, fashion and music rapidly became more corporate, drugs more ruinous, hypocrisy more blatant—and prosperity's basis in cheap oil exposed and compromised. Prior successes had been predicated on a seemingly endless and undamaging supply of cheap energy and the ongoing preparedness of corporations to share the profits of the labor and material they controlled with (some of) their First World employees. Once oil prices leapt following cartel action from the Global South in 1973, unemployment and inflation soared across the Global North. In retrospect, it is clear that Western Europe and the United States were, ironically, oil states, in that their domestic and international political power relied on it.[18]

It was a sad time to be young and have imagined oneself part of a coming generation of change in Britain. A new discourse wiped away the postwar settlement between capital and labor, the currency was devalued, and the International Monetary Fund (IMF) was invited to assist. A racialized law-and-order discourse grew in strength, while progressive social movements such as feminism and Black and gay power suffered White-male intransigence and economic chaos.[19]

I experienced a shift from Swinging London to postimperial decrepitude via endless rain, unremitting damp, and a persistently dull yet fundamentally untrustworthy world. For those of us studying during a three-day week, with darkness folding in from 4 p.m. until 8 a.m., reading and writing via gaslight, TV broadcasts ending early, shivering temperatures, misery abounding, Piccadilly thrown into darkness, collieries closed, politics a shamble, toilet paper in short supply, and teeth cleaned in the gloom, 1973 marked the fifth state of emergency declared in three years. Then the millennial occupation of Ireland brought its first major blowback as bombing came to Britain.

Unbeknownst to the likes of me, the United Kingdom had hidden economic strengths: a colonial inheritance of overseas investments, which brought in untold riches, and an appeal for the wealthy and connected of the Global South as a place where their children would not be kidnapped or their power questioned. The country was ceasing to be a colonist, a quarry, and a farm and starting a new life as a depository, a safe house for the global elite in an emergent neoliberal order.

I was also often in the United States during the mid-1970s, where an unremitting pessimism was equally all consuming. The country's unparalleled sense of economic, military, and constitutional superiority was challenged if not subdued by the oil crisis, Watergate, Vietnam, and urban revolt, not to mention a "stream of disclosure about covert counterinsurgency in every form, from secretly underwritten academic research to assassinations and mass killings."[20] At the same time, its extraordinary influence on world affairs was unabated.

The United States, too, was making a transition from being a quarry, farm, and factory to a copyright and finance economy, a model of structural adjustment for the Global North (until it went too far and jeopardized manufacturing). In Mexico, the discovery of sizeable new oil reserves and accession to the Organisation for Economic Co-operation and Development (OECD) were quickly followed by economic disaster, while Colombia saw a deepening conflict between the government and various guerrilla forces and intensified narco violence as the needy nostrils of the North feathered demand.

There was a sense of disaster throughout the First World, of rising unemployment and inflation, of booming interest rates, of failed generational change. Capital took this as an opportunity for governmental action to control wage increases and redistribute wealth upward. It has been thus ever since. For five decades, the ensuing neoliberal ideology has underpinned economic policy in most of the world, further stimulated by the waning of state socialism in Eastern and Central Europe from 1989 and the emergence of a massive reserve army of labor in the People's Republic of China (PRC) since 2000, when the global pool of workers virtually doubled overnight.[21]

How was this intellectual/policy transformation achieved, and how does it reproduce itself? Through a theory that manufactures a fantastical version of truth that it then makes real by influencing public policy and populist propaganda. Pierre

Bourdieu's cuttingly astringent words disclose the lies that underpin this fakery. He asks, "Is the economic world really, as the dominant discourse would have us believe, a pure and perfect order" or rather "the implementation of a utopia, neo-liberalism, thus converted into a political programme" that is presented "as the scientific description of reality?"[22]

In the history of philosophy, the possibility of truth has often been clear. Uncovering it was not easy but unquestionably desirable. It was largely essayed via two models. Correspondence theories aimed to present rather than represent information, with no mediation between knowledge and people other than external corroboration in the world. Coherence theories assumed the implausibility of a perfect match between truth and understanding, so they depended on a consistent and transparent intellectual method that permitted the replication of claims.[23]

We all know the grand, yet purportedly antigrand, narrative of the 1980s and 1990s that intersected with neoliberalism and questioned those logics—the postmodern. It originated as a set of bracing intellectual, artistic, and architectural movements but encouraged the widespread and profound rejection of expertise.[24] Hitherto dominant means of establishing the truth were deemed to be compromised. Science, history, religion, and philosophy lost credibility due to their long-standing service in support of imperialism, slavery, colonialism, capitalism, Marxism-Leninism, fascism, Maoism, misogyny, inequality, war, and poverty.[25]

In their place came the *différend*. Certain modes of speech were deemed to be so comprehensively incommensurate with one another that no means of deciding between them could do so without violating their respective codes of communication.[26] The magical denial of this irreconcilability became the ultimate force of myth: ignoring one's conditions of existence to pronounce on, or force to cohere, fundamentally opposed genres of speech. Everything became contingent and multiperspectival. The two delineable phases of truth and lies grew indistinct. With underlying reality lost and rigorous norms cast aside, signs became self-referential, with no residual correspondence to the real: they adopted the form of their own simulation.[27]

Neoliberal ideas emerged into that vacuum of social, economic, and theoretical uncertainty. They did not thrive thanks to an inherent rightness or popular appeal, though they provide a veneer of coherence.[28] Rather, neoliberalism has been popularized by the movement's intellectual minions, who indulge in a "permanent criticism of government policy"[29] that defines and measures itself as a counter to Keynesianism. They bloviate against expertise (for populism), against subvention (for markets), and against public service (for philanthropy).[30] The doctrine's core putative commitments are individualism, consumerism, property rights, opposition to trade unionism, reduced tariffs, and minimal democratic regulation of industries: "Licensing capital, leashing labor, demonizing the social state and the political, attacking equality, promulgating freedom."[31]

Neoliberalism holds that comparative advantage in global competition must inform economic policy based on countries' particular factor endowments of climate, terrain, finance, and workforce. Its ideologists call for the state to generate more and more markets with fewer and fewer democratic controls, insist on limiting the cost of supply (i.e., wages), and deride governments as sources of demand. They celebrate that whereas "the initial postwar decades witnessed exploding socialism, followed by creeping or stagnant socialism . . . the pressure today is toward giving markets a greater role and government a smaller one."[32]

These organic intellectuals of the ruling class have similar tactics, arguments, and financing as the tobacco lobby in its long-standing assault on public health. Adopting the cloak of "merchants of doubt," they peddle hundreds of millions of dollars to fend off anticapitalist scientific findings.[33] Key chorines of neoliberal shibboleths include such coin-operated think tanks as the Mercatus Center, the Centre for Policy Studies, the American Enterprise Institute, the Committee for a Constructive Tomorrow, the Fundación Naumann para la Libertad, the George C. Marshall Institute, the Global Warming Policy Foundation, the Club de la Libertad de Corrientes, the Acton Institute, the Judicial Crisis Network, the Heartland Institute, the Claremont Institute, the Legatum Institute, the Fundación Internacional Bases, the Science and Public Policy Institute, the Discovery Institute, the Manhattan Institute for Policy Research, the Lavoisier Group, the Leadership Institute, the Hoover Institution, Fundación Eléutera, the Institute for Public Affairs, the Vivekananda International Foundation, the Centre for Independent Studies, the Instituto Mises, the Fundación Pensar, the Institut Économique Molinari, the Reason Foundation, the Institute of Economic Affairs, the Latin America Liberty Forum, the Fraser Institute, the Business Environmental Leadership Council, the Movimiento Brasil Libre, the India Foundation, the TaxPayers' Alliance, the John Locke Foundation, the Council for National Policy, the Cato Institute, the Syama Prasad Mookerjee Research Foundation, the Menzies Research Centre, the Family Research Council, the Heritage Foundation, the American Enterprise Institute, the World Business Council on Sustainable Development, the Ludwig von Mises Institute, the Europäisches Institut für Klima und Energie, the Initiative for Free Trade, the Instituto Juan de Mariana, the E Foundation for Oklahoma, the Public Policy Research

Centre, Open Europe, the Cobden Centre, the Charles Koch Foundation, the Club for Growth, the Adam Smith Institute, the Liberales Institut, Estudiantes por la Libertad, the India Policy Foundation, FreedomWorks, the Mont Pelerin Society, and the Competitive Enterprise Institute, inter alia.[34] Many are part of a loose global group known as the Atlas Network.[35] So imposing. So euphemistic.[36]

Many of these organizations hire people with doctorates, include faculty members as affiliates, and couch their self-dealing in scholarly terms. Dozens of volumes appear that deny or welcome climate change—virtually none written by qualified authors or subjected to adequate review. Such "research" feeds op-eds in newspapers and talking points on cable news, where a noxious blend of corporate self-interest, religious superstition, and public manipulation delivers snatched column inches and shouted seconds to overworked, underresourced journalists. Angry yet oddly supine swivel-heads feast on minor disagreements among climate or syndemic experts, which are mendaciously misconstrued as evidence that the relevant science is fraudulent.[37] The companies that fund this duplicity sometimes go further, rebranding themselves as stakeholders in the green economy and even promoting sustainability and capitalism as natural partners.[38] Dutifully obeying the données of an imaginary neoliberal world, they argue that once prices are placed on such negative externalities as pollution, everything will be put to rights through the operation of supply and demand.[39]

Given the fervor accompanying this extraordinary self-anointed claim to omniscience and omnipotence, it comes as no surprise that neoclassical economics has religious origins. When the Trinity was being ideologized within Christianity, something had to be done to legitimize the concept as well as dismiss and decry polytheistic and pagan rivals to the new religion's moralistic monotheism. To resolve this problem, sacerdotes invented *oikonomia*, a sphere of worldly arrangements that was to be directed by a physical presence on Earth who could represent the will of the deity. God gave Christ "the economy" to manage, so "the economy" indexically manifested Christianity.[40] Like religion, neoliberal lust for market conduct extends to a passion for comprehending and opining on everything from birth rates to divorce, from suicide to abortion, and from performance-enhancing drugs to altruism—rarely if ever referring to theories or research from beyond its own cozy barrio.[41]

Hence Margaret Hilda Thatcher's certainty that "we have gone through a period when too many children and people have been given to understand 'I have a problem, it is the Government's job to cope with it!' or 'I have a problem, I will go and get a grant to cope with it!' 'I am homeless, the Government must house me!' and so they are casting their problems on society and who is society? There is no such thing!"[42] Here is her disciple, the Conservative Party's then secretary of state for social security, Peter Bruce Lilley, promising to "close down the something-for-nothing society" as he regaled the party's 1992 annual conference with this ditty borrowed from *The Mikado*:

> I've got a little list / Of benefit offenders who I'll soon be rooting out / And who never would be missed / They never would be missed. / There's those who make up bogus claims / In half a dozen names / And councillors who draw the dole / To run left-wing campaigns / They never would be missed / They never would be missed. / There's young ladies who get pregnant just to jump the housing queue / And dads who won't support the kids / of ladies they have . . . kissed / And I haven't even mentioned all those sponging socialists / I've got them on my list / And there's none of them be missed / There's none of them be missed.[43]

This embrace of neoliberal cruelty was met with rapturous applause. He's now a baron.

Such denials of real life, and knowledge of it, reached their rhetorical apogee in 2003, when Mexican president Vicente Fox Quesada asked reporters, "¿Yo por qué? . . . ¿Qué no somos 100 millones de mexicanos?" (Why me? . . . Aren't there a hundred million Mexicans?).[44] In other words, each person must assume responsibility for his or her material fortunes. The fact that not every one of the other hundred million Mexicans exercised control over the country's money supply, tariff policy, trade, labor law, public health, education, security, and exchange rate might have given him pause. Or not. And Thatcher of course "left the British state, more powerful, and more concentrated" than she found it; "an authoritarian state was necessary to support markets controlled by corporations and banks."[45]

The idea that neoliberalism represents a return to a state of nature, where markets adjudicate life by adjusting a mystical equilibrium, is misleading. Rather, it attempts to create "an enterprise society" through the boring but efficaciously virile pretense that the latter is an organic state of affairs, even as competition is imposed as a framework for regulating everyday life via a subtly comprehensive statism. The idea is to manufacture ratiocinative liberal actors while proclaiming them to be the work of nature. The competitive market is neoliberalism's privileged "interface of government and the individual," the latter internalizing laissez-faire criteria as a constellation of habits, choices, disgusts, delights, and judgments expressed as characteristics of personal identity.[46] Demagogues plead for investments in human capital while deriding government-led social engineering. They hail "freedom" as a natural basis for life—provided they can employ the heavy hand of policing to administer property relations and preclude democratic intervention into capitalism. In short, neoliberalism seeks to govern all things while opposing democratic control of them.

The purportedly disruptive economic trends lauded by these people are not due to much-vaunted capitalist innovation or market adjustment but to scholarly advances and taxpayer risk-taking. One example is the cell phone, a key tool of public health in the syndemic. Touted by neoliberals as the outcome and stimulant of unfettered market forces and creativity,[47] it is nothing of the kind. If we lift the lid on today's smartphones, what do we find? Click wheels, multitouch screens, Global Positioning Systems, lithium-ion batteries, signal compression, hypertext markup language, liquid-crystal displays, and so on. Did those elements, so neatly combined by the corporations whose names and icons are emblazoned inside our jackets and pocketbooks, emerge via the magic of laissez-faire from a desire to compete with one another to meet consumers' needs? No. These donations to corporate profits came from the U.S. Defense Advanced Research Projects Agency, the European Organization for Nuclear Research, the U.S. Department of Energy, the CIA, the National Science Foundation, the U.S. Navy, the U.S. Army Research Office, the National Institutes of Health, the U.S. Department of Defense, the European Organization for Nuclear Research, and universities that did their bidding.[48]

The real deal is that as each element of Keynesian demand management has unraveled in the name of privatization and deregulation, neoliberals have revealed themselves to be at the heart of state projects, aided by researchers in more scholarly fields. Why do the latter go along with this?

Apart from material gain and prestige, the answer may lie with the left-wing nuclear scientists who were so crucial to the Manhattan Project. Testifying before the U.S. Atomic Energy Commission in the 1950s, Julius Robert Oppenheimer, who led the group that developed the bomb, talked about the instrumental rationality that animated his colleagues. Once they saw what was scientifically and monetarily feasible, the device's murderous impact lost intellectual and emotional significance for them—overtaken by what he called its "technically sweet" quality.[49]

Such saccharine is the lifeblood of a technological sublime, but as Oppenheimer showed in retrospect, even its closest adherents may sometimes step outside their immediate circumstances and pleasures to provide us with critical insights into the emotional appeal that can underpin instrumental rationality. For Marx, recognizing oneself as a species can generate class consciousness over consumer sovereignty and expand that awareness to encompass other forms of life—albeit too late, in this case.[50] We shall see what happened when COVID scientists came to such a realization.

Militaristic links between research and capitalism have a history prior even to the dread hand of neoliberalism overreaching itself. In his farewell speech as U.S. president at the birth of the 1960s, former Supreme Commander of the Allied Expeditionary Force in Europe, President of Columbia University, and lifelong dutiful Republican Dwight David Eisenhower memorably condemned "the military-industrial complex."[51] He was referring to the cozy relationships between the men running the military and the armaments industries. Those relationships were forged by class, gender, race, education, militarism, and warfare welfare.

Eisenhower was speaking at the height of the Cold War, when mutual disrespect, misunderstanding, ignorance, and aggression characterized the U.S.-U.S.S.R. relationship. He knew how silly the massive military expenditure of both nations was—that it was leading their societies toward misdirected, bloated budgets of violence and angry, anxious people. But that would supposedly end once "we" had won.

Thirty years ago, the Cold War ended. This "we" duly awaited a peace dividend. Much of the world's mad and maddening expenditure on violence could be redirected away from the military-industrial complex Eisenhower had so presciently described and toward social services and the Global South.[52]

It didn't happen.

The amount that wealthy countries continue to spend on "defense" shows how right he was about the enduring power of the military-industrial complex and how deleterious it would be for economies and societies.[53] In 2015, 39 percent of U.S. income tax went to military institutions, underwriting soldiers, colleges, and corporations—our welfare royalty.[54] If only it had gone to the environment, education, and health care for all. Across the Global North, warfare remained resilient against neoliberal critiques of taxation.

But that dominant discourse proved remarkably effective at eviscerating valuable public expenditure and surviving even the 2008 financial crisis. It rocked neoliberalism around the world because deregulated financial sectors collapsed under the weight of their manifold contradictions. Charles Ferguson's 2010 documentary, *Inside Job*,[55] and associated research exposed the fact that leading economists opined on the public interest before, during, and after pocketing hefty sitting and speaking fees as corporate consultants and conference lounge lizards.[56] But the brute ideology survived, so great were the investments in it by intellectuals, corporations, states, and international organizations. The crisis it had created was resolved via a familiar formula: socialism for the wealthy and capitalism for the poor.[57] Huge bailouts of major capitalist enterprises by governments—something supposedly antithetical to neoliberals—restored the system, plunging treasuries into debt and legitimizing subsequent reductions in social services, coupled with tax hikes for ordinary people. Bankers were bankrolled, homeowners evicted, accountants acquitted, and neoclassical economists pardoned (by themselves). Neoliberal tentacles continue to control much of ordinary life and policymaking; *Dead Ideas Still Walk among Us*.[58] They are the latest bulwark to elitist tendencies that lie at the heart of capital.

Almost a century ago, F. Scott Fitzgerald penned these famous words in his short story "The Rich Boy":

> Let me tell you about the very rich. They are different from you and me. They possess and enjoy early, and it does something to them, makes them soft where we are hard, and cynical where we are trustful, in a way that, unless you were born rich, it is very difficult to understand. They think, deep in their hearts, that they are better than we are because we had to discover the compensations and refuges of life for ourselves. Even when they enter deep into our world or sink below us, they still think that they are better than we are. They are different.[59]

A decade later, Ernest Hemingway wrote the following in "The Snows of Kilimanjaro" ("Julian" stood in for Fitzgerald in the story, after the real-life author had reacted badly to being named directly in an earlier version.[60]):

> The rich were dull and they drank too much, or they played too much backgammon. They were dull and they were repetitious. He remembered poor Julian and his romantic awe of them and how he had started a story once that began, "The very rich are different from you and me." And how someone had said to Julian, Yes, they have more money. But that was not humorous to Julian. He thought they were a

special glamourous race and when he found they weren't it
wrecked him just as much as any other thing
that wrecked him.[61]

There's a reason we still read these deeply flawed, arrogant, self-satisfied, tortured, and torturing critics and fans of U.S. life. It's not just to do with their clipped, clear prose and reporters' eyes.[62] Fitzgerald and Hemingway may not have disabused their readers of a belief in the dollar transcending the class privilege that leading populists are, ironically, so often born into. But they found a way to ask what differentiated those with real, unearned power from the rest of us—especially folks who place their faith in demagogic pronouncements. Fitzgerald and Hemingway understood how oligarchs and oligopolists comport themselves. And their words ring true for the United Kingdom, Colombia, and Mexico as well.

How we need them now.

When I asked the editor of a glossy magazine for the superwealthy how his subscribers were responding to the 2008 crisis and what impact it was having on advertising revenues, he replied, "They don't know there's a crisis. And advertising is holding up just fine, thank you." He turned firmly on his Southern Californian heel while his girlfriend urged me to buy her new self-help book. I imagine life still goes on for his readers, even if they may worry a wee bit nowadays about home delivery. But not too, too much. After all, the research tells us that the wealthier U.S. people are, the less they empathize with others' suffering and the more contempt they show for the poor.[63]

Lamentably, the public gets little help from bourgeois journalism in understanding the dominant discourse's falsehoods and its winners and victims. Journalism should play a pivotal role in sharing the scientific, social, and political information upon which public understanding of the environment, health, and the economy depends.[64] The idea is to draw citizens into the policy process, ensuring informed public comment and dissent as well as willing consent. It relies on adequate resources to permit research, interpretation, and dissemination.

Regrettably, hypercommercialization of the news and disinvestment in investigative research have diminished public trust in reporters and their capacity to counter distortions.[65] The deregulation of the media has cultivated the birth and maturation, if that's the right word, of neoliberalism's postmodern and populist cousins: post-truth and fake news. Journalism is frequently just one more industrial process ruled by dominant economic forces that reduce ideological or generic innovation in favor of standardization. The spread of "fake" news through churnalism and unscrupulous trolls has become a topic for tweets and inquiries from the Oval Office, the U.K. Parliament, EU headquarters, and everywhere in between.[66] The Oxford Dictionary's Word of the Year for 2016 was *post-truth*: "relating to or denoting circumstances in which objective facts are less influential in shaping public opinion than appeals to emotion and personal belief."[67] For all its origins in knowing postmodern satire, fake news will forever be associated with 2016: Britain's referendum on Brexit, the Colombian plebiscite on peace, and the U.S. general elections. In each case, public opinion was manipulated by international and national reactionaries, from covert to overt forces, from Russian espionage to gringo evangelism.[68]

A coordinated assault on expertise by right-wing populism is the latest and most important index of what has been jeopardized and lost thanks to a cheery, self-confident questioning of formal knowledge; the assiduous discrediting of anthropological, sociological, and historical work;

and a touching cybertarian faith that the newer media will return us to Eden, an imaginary world of innocence and pure communication.[69] Although neoliberalism survived 2008, technocracy was profoundly imperiled because of its signal failure during boom times to aid the working class—and signal determination to blame and tax it when crisis set in. The upshot was organic intellectuals like Donald John Trump (I know, it hurts to read that) and Brexit demagogues exploiting a wave of anger.[70]

Craziness has taken hold across the terrain of social life, perhaps nowhere more crucially than in public health. Whenever there is a fiscal crisis, as per 2008, risk is socialized and wealth privatized.[71] More and more people in Mexico, Colombia, the United States, and Britain acknowledge that a meritocracy is unattainable and inequality unfair, but there is no serious political alternative on offer.[72] As a consequence, many turn to the angry, frustrated sounds of squealing ruling-class scions whose affected common touch offers an array of figures to be blamed for social ills—intellectuals, experts, city dwellers, racial minorities, feminists, journalists, Hollywood actors, and immigrants.[73]

We've seen a tide of such ignorance, arrogance, bigotry, and irresponsibility flood the airwaves and internet, courtesy of cunning simpletons housed in DC, Mexico City, Brasilia, and London (Trump, Andrés Manuel López Obrador, Jair Messias Bolsonaro, and Alexander Boris de Pfeffel Johnson). The special brand of intellectual underachievement that characterizes their governmental maladministration has been matched by the discipleship of their gullible followers—and the service they provide to smarter, but equally selfish, capital. In the United States' case, this has been exacerbated by decades of direct and indirect corporate funding propagandizing about the role of Christianity in founding the nation. These attacks on secularism and the state date from opposition to the New Deal through to the present. They are tied to the Republican Party's Southern strategy, adopted in 1968 in reaction to the civil rights movement. It associates the allegedly willful misuse of welfare with minorities and creates a voting bloc identified with White evangelism and against Blackness.[74] Bankrolled by companies and individuals keen on neoliberal policies and prepared to exploit demagogues, these tendencies have been remarkably effective. In Colombia, which has been run by technocrats who are more rational and hence have lower profiles, the same process has applied but without the asinine hysteria. President Iván Duque Márquez spent many years at the Inter-American Development Bank. Unlike the premiers listed above, he knows how to appear rational and reasonable but pursues policies akin to the populists who supposedly eschew his insider politics. Oligarchs and oligopolists sleep tight with such men securing their interests.

To set matters straight, we need a political-economic approach, for the material outcomes of neoliberal hegemony are abysmal, as the four nations I examine show—amply and tragically. And whereas we used to query big science's faith in unconditional truth, today we must endorse its piecemeal labors toward comprehending COVID.

The Record

In the United States, the capacity to exit poverty has diminished over the last five decades, thanks to a gigantic clumping of wealth among the few. They sit atop the many, who are poor, unskilled, and unhealthy. Tens of millions of U.S. residents are indigent, functionally analphabetic, and lacking any or adequate health care—the highest proportions in the Global North. Thirty million have no health insurance. The number of working-class people reporting extreme distress has tripled over the last three decades, almost always associated with unemployment. As productivity and profit have risen, ordinary people's purchasing power has plummeted. Inequality is at Depression levels. In the three years prior to 2020, life expectancy fell for the first time since the 1918 influenza.[75] We're moving backward, arching toward a history that reinstates the worst of secondary accumulation.

Forty years ago, the nation's credulous, sedulous neoclassical economists hailed the impact of market precepts over Western European social democracy because just 20 percent of the U.S. public's future income was predictable based on paternal income. By the 1990s, and two more decades of deregulation, that figure had doubled. Some suggest it now stands at 60 percent. In the two decades since 1979, the highest-paid 1 percent of the population doubled its share of national pretax income, to 18 percent. The incomes of the top 1 percent increased by 194 percent, the top 20 percent by 70 percent, and the bottom 20 percent by just 6.4 percent. In 1967, chief executive officers of corporations were paid twenty-four times the average wage of employees. Thirty years later, they received three hundred times that amount.[76]

Half the money made by capital goes to a tenth of the population, even as tax burdens shift dramatically from companies to workers. If we juxtapose aggregate prosperity against personal insecurity, the economy is doing well by ruling-class indices but poorly by proletarian ones, both in terms of inequality and instability.[77] The gap between what labor produces and what it reaps is greater now than at any point since the advent of working-class electoral franchises.[78] Had the national growth in income between 1975 and 2018 been shared as it was in the 1950s and '60s, earnings "for the population below the 90th percentile over this time period would have been $2.5 trillion (67 percent) higher in 2018."[79] And the neoliberal era has produced an explosion of "multidimensional poverty" through food insecurity, poor education, and insufficient health care.[80]

Britain has seen a similar deepening of inequality, over the same period, underpinned by the same ideology. And like the United States, this has occurred on a bipartisan basis. Nominally worker-oriented parties—Labour in the United Kingdom, the Democrats in the United States—have presided over catastrophic triumphs of capital as merrily as have the avowed parties of business, respectively the Conservatives and Republicans. Whereas supposedly social-democratic tendencies were formerly associated with working-class, minimally educated voters, their electoral base has shifted to people with high levels of cultural capital. William Jefferson Clinton and Anthony Charles Lynton Blair, Barack Hussein Obama II and David William Donald Cameron—the difference has made no difference.[81] Meanwhile, the regime of tax cuts over which they and their kind presided has remorselessly, predictably, stimulated monumental inequality while doing nothing—nothing—for employment.[82]

Between 1980 and 2017, Britain's gross domestic product (GDP) shot up by 100 percent. Impressive. But that didn't come close to the growth in the number of its food banks—1000 percent.[83] Employment reached record levels, as did the number of employees living in poverty and receiving less and less welfare support.[84] The United Kingdom boasts the worst sick pay provisions in the Global North and a drastically crumbling and disappearing infrastructure, from youth clubs to parks to pubs to libraries.[85] A secondary labor market is in play. On the cusp of the coronavirus, 14.5 million lived in poverty—more than one in every five people. The key sufferers were private and social renters, residents of areas with high unemployment, single parents, minorities, and freelancers.[86]

Latin America provides another example of the devastation wrought by this brutal reconsolidation of elite parthenogenesis. The region had pursued nationalist/Keynesian projects of import-substitution industrialization from the 1930s through the 1970s.[87] But neoliberalism's recipe for economic and social development in the Global South is export-oriented industrialization: sell your best coffee, avocado, oil, quinoa, and tequila overseas; don't set up your own automobile company or airline. For fifty years, financial institutions and international organizations have dished out punishments for investing in welfare or "anachronistic" economic policies.

Obediently following northern fashion, Latin America has deregulated and privatized, satisfying domestic oligarchs and northern masters alike.[88] Today, the region stands ready to meet the rich world's needs by guaranteeing environmental despoliation, clientelism, and brutal labor-market restructuring in place of guaranteed income, agrarian reform, free health care, and public education K through college.[89]

A deregulatory intellectual logic has prevailed. Elites have sent their "brightest" sons and daughters to U.S. graduate school for indoctrination into the happy world of factor endowments, monetarism, dedemocratization, and anti-Marxism.[90] From Washington to Yale and back again, self-serving, self-dealing, next-generation Colombian and Mexican scions have purred along with the pride of northern neoliberal lions.[91] On return, these children of the oligarchy assume positions of enormous influence, forwarding "policy-based evidence" while claiming to be animated by "evidence-based policy."[92] Duque is an exemplar. The upshot of that history? Poverty across the region is skyrocketing. It is predicted to number 231 million people shortly—a level not seen for years.[93]

Colombia and Mexico both show the lineaments of their tumultuous invasion and independence and the systematic inequality forged from that unique history.[94] Each is dogged by powerful political, economic, and cultural oligarchies and oligopolies; manifest, manifold corruption; intense and unremitting racism operating within the ideology of *mestizaje* (hybridity); profound religiosity, be it Catholic or Evangelical; and the forever looming, forbidding, inciting, prescribing, proscribing, and above all, intervening presence of the United States.[95] The long-standing and contemporary reality of a nation at war with itself for eight decades, at the cost of hundreds of thousands murdered and millions displaced, is that Colombians view their country as a profoundly corrupt blend of collusive private and public interests, clientelism, limited state authority, fraudulent elections, and criminal-justice abuses. Mexicans regard their long history of authoritarian populism very similarly.[96]

Despite lengthy economic growth, and virtually zero inflation, Colombia has half its people living below the poverty line, compared to a third in 1980. The nation's elite received a fifth of all national income between 1990 and 2010.[97] The richest 10 percent of the population is four times wealthier than the poorest 40 percent. Under the current administration, corporate taxes and surcharges have plunged from 40 percent to 33 percent, and regressive indirect taxation has soared to 19 percent.[98] OXFAM estimates that "over 67 percent of productive land is concentrated in 0.4 percent of agricultural landholdings."[99] Together with this misallocation of wealth and a neoliberal economic model based on extractivism, corruption makes Colombia the most unequal country in Latin America and the seventh in the world.[100]

The Mexican story is similar: 10 percent of families hold 70 percent of the nation's wealth, with just 1 percent controlling 40 percent of the money.[101] Social policies have been aimed at a minority of the labor force—people employed in conventional waged and salaried jobs—largely to the exclusion of the informal sector. The requirement to pay levies to fund welfare encourages businesses and workers alike to function informally, which in turn reduces consolidated revenue and hence governmental funds for education and other services.[102]

Inevitably and inexorably, neoliberal dogma aids the wealthy at the expense of the poor. Waves of fixed capital formation investment and contraction cycle with international demand for commodities. Public works are undertaken to enable capital or manage environmental catastrophes. These policies slow growth, boost the informal sector, and generate ever-greater inequality through unemployment, underemployment, and disinvestment in social security systems. Local and visiting oligarchs benefit from such policy shibboleths alongside, shall we say, "discretionary" commitments to legality.[103] In both Colombia and Mexico, cocaine, violence, and neoliberalism have followed "a model and a mythology of development whilst waging a phony war on drugs and drug dealers who have been incorporated into, and/or deployed by, elites in their genuine wars to dispossess rural citizens."[104]

Especially bloody conflicts have catalyzed across deregulated mining, agribusiness, and tourism. More environmental defenders in the region were killed over the last decade and a half than the number of British and Australian soldiers lost in imperial U.S. wars.[105] Many more were tossed into jail or threatened. All dared to question rapacious land use by the extractive industries. They became victims of a vicious amalgam of the military, contract assassins, and private security forces.[106] Meanwhile, new fractions of capital exploited the financial sector's invention of monetary instruments to launder their plunder.[107]

I suppose that's what neoliberal prelates mean when they incant "innovation."

Health

Health care varies massively, expensively, and conflictually across states, regions, and the globe.[108] The present moment sees numerous major players jostling for position to deal with and profit from COVID-19. The PRC, the United States, Russia, and the EU have large populations, immense economic power, international ambitions, and vested interests, notably those of large pharmaceutical corporations and complicit research infrastructures.

How might we understand the prevailing health conjuncture in geopolitical terms? Two forms of thought suggest themselves. One is the realist theory of international relations, which proposes that most key struggles in world politics are decided by the wealthiest and most militarily powerful actors.[109] The other is political-economic theory. It veers away from an exclusive focus on the world of states and associated methodological nationalism to examine the powerful multinational corporations headquartered within their boundaries as well as domestic and foreign oligarchs and oligopolies.[110] We can see the value of both approaches in the ongoing struggle for economic and military hegemony between the PRC and the United States and the impact of that conflict across the globe. Such macho posturing has colored the syndemic crisis, especially with the ongoing tendency to refuse the legitimacy of international organizations, most notably the World Health Organization (WHO).

Here's the U.S. history that shows how dependent capitalist health care is on the state and how it fails to serve the people in whose name it justifies its existence.

Bulk buying of medicines during the Civil War encouraged both profits and professionalization. The U.S. federal government proceeded to create the business conditions that eventually generated pharmaceutical corporations. They received further stimulus from the Great War through the mass purchase of aspirin and patent-breaking treatments for syphilis. In response to addiction, regulations mandated prescriptions for several drugs from 1914, further institutionalizing the power of large firms and the medical profession. An emergent big pharma mounted scientific research and management, while doctors profited from increased visits by patients in search of medicines. Then the United States "liberated" discoveries from the advanced pharmaceutical industries of a defeated Germany after the Second World War. In 1951, the federal government mandated that all new medicines be subject to prescription. This marked both a grab for professional standards and control and a new form of commodity production.[111]

The pharmaceutical industry's proportion of U.S. health research grew from 13 percent in 1980 to 52 percent in 1995. But marketing, not science, determines how to develop a new medicinal compound once it has been uncovered, asking such questions as Will this be promoted as a counter to depression or ejaculation? Will it be announced in journal *x* or *y*? and Which scholars will be chosen to front the new drug and produce consensus over its benefits? Major advertising agencies provide ghostwriting services, funded by pharma, that deliver copy to academics and clinicians—then pay them for signing it. Faculty who shill for corporations put their names to articles they have neither researched nor written. There are few if any concessions to conflicts of interest, let alone public declarations of this cash-for-research-and-comment love fest. One in ten papers published in leading medical outlets across the 1990s were the work of ghosts.

An astounding 90 percent of *Journal of the American Medical Association* articles that decade were "authored" by people paid by pharmacorps, which also pressured journals to print favorable findings in return for lucrative advertising copy.[112] Such revelations have led the International Committee of Medical Journal Editors to investigate who does the research and writing that its members publish.[113]

In addition, pseudoscholars from medical schools and professional practice groups routinely accept monetary and travel gifts from companies as *quae pro quibus* for favorable publicity.[114] Novartis funded more than a third of the activities of the Plant Biology Department at Berkeley between 1998 and 2003. When a faculty member who criticized this arrangement was denied tenure, external reviewers found the decision was influenced by the prevailing political economy.[115] It's all part of *Science-Mart*, where applied knowledge is corrupted by corporate and university desire.[116] Belated efforts at legislation have nevertheless allowed key shapers of opinion to continue on their merry way as creatures of big pharma.[117]

Meanwhile, clientelist politicians readily serve health corporations. Consider the double-declutching of ex-Representative James Greenwood, who shifted ever so easily, ever so directly from chairing a House subcommittee charged with monitoring pharmaceuticals to running the splendidly named Biotechnology Innovation Organization, a lobby group for firms he had supposedly just been interrogating, such as Pfizer, Bristol Myers Squibb, Eli Lilly, and GlaxoSmithKline. Together, they work assiduously to beat back legislative efforts that might curb their superprofits. As a consequence, prices for medical drugs in the United States are higher than the Global North norm.[118] Party on, dude. And as the health industries grab more and more slices of GDP, beyond anything imaginable elsewhere, medicine is practiced under the sign of insurance surveillance, dominated by treatment parameters rather than actual care. All this arose and continues as a consequence of political lobbying by interested parties—excluding patients. That's the *Public Creation of the Corporate Health System*.[119]

There has been some change: a vast array of health maintenance organizations (HMOs) has undermined previously hegemonic powerbrokers through a discourse of bureaucratic-managerial commodification. Since the advent of wholesale managed care versus fee-for-service in the mid-1990s, insurance-company support for doctor-patient interaction has declined: HMOs want to reduce long-term, face-to-face, and inpatient treatment.[120]

The upshot is that the United States has the most inefficient, expensive, and technologically competent health care in the world, its reform stymied by insurance firms lobbying in the purported name of individual choice. In Robert Reich's sober but frustrated words, we have a "private for-profit system for individuals lucky enough to afford it and a rickety social insurance system for people fortunate enough to have a full-time job."[121] A third of workers, three-quarters of whom are on low wages, lack any entitlement to paid sick leave.[122] Prior to the syndemic, twenty-eight million citizens had no health insurance, and fifteen million soon lost employer coverage along with their jobs.[123] Adding to the poverty trap and institutional failings, many health-care professionals have long shown a preference for White patients over minorities.[124]

By contrast, Britain's socialized National Health Service (NHS) does function for the vast majority of its citizens. The NHS began after the war, following a decade of worthy lobbying and planning from the Socialist Medical Association and the exemplar of the Welsh Tredegar Workmen's Medical Aid Society. In the possibly mythic words of Aneurin

Bevan, the politician forever associated with the advent of the NHS, "Illness should neither be an indulgence for which people have to pay, nor an offence for which they should be penalised, but a misfortune, the cost of which should be shared by the community."[125] You know, socialism. It was part of a raft of postwar reforms designed to ameliorate poverty and ensure a functioning labor force.[126]

Given low life expectancy, the notion was that health care and pensions would be neither extensive nor expensive. The NHS would quickly fix recoverable maladies that affected workers and cut costs for the wealthy. But with new drugs and increased public-health awareness, life expectancy rose, as did the cost of the NHS. Along with it came popular approval, to the point where public health became akin to social security in the United States—a beloved part of life, albeit one subject to a covert and malevolent privatization that began with contracting out cleaning services in the early 1980s to firms hiring schoolchildren. Unsurprisingly, ward infections skyrocketed. Ever since, the NHS has been progressively distorted and defanged by bipartisan attempts to control and pauperize it through capitalistic methods of scientific management/Taylorism and reduced purchasing power.[127] It reached the point even prior to the syndemic where critical care was, so to speak, in critical condition.[128]

In Latin America, the last three decades have seen a dutiful, disastrous marketization of health care. The result? A third of medical expenditure is paid for out of pocket.[129] Mexico's system instantiates class divisions in both public and private sectors. The former is bifurcated between indigent citizens of the informal economy and those with conventional jobs that carry with them contributions toward national insurance. Total expenditure on health care meets barely half the benchmarks set by the Pan American Health Organization (PAHO) and the OECD.[130] The number of hospital beds per thousand people has diminished dramatically over the last decade to 0.98, and the ratio of physicians has dropped from 2.9 in 2005 to 2.4.[131] A new system for those working in the informal sector was put in place for 2020 but has been underfunded and problematically administered.[132] Private medical services require payment at the time of service. They are rapid and technologized, to the point where medical tourism from the Global North is rife among both temporarily returning nationals and gringos in search of high-quality, cheap care.[133]

Over the last three decades, Colombia has "reformed" health care predicated on the belief that capital can operate more efficiently and effectively than the state, thereby maximizing coverage and minimizing inequality of access and utilization of health services. In reality, there are "raging inequities within Colombia's health-care system, which has been lauded for providing near-universal coverage but widely criticized for providing dramatically inferior care to the less affluent."[134]

A model of managed competition has seen hospitals compete to sell their wares and become freestanding businesses. In place of the demand subsidies that assisted patients directly in the past, they receive supply subsidies from the state. The system has dual insurance plans: a contributory one, which is mandatorily funded by public and private employees in the formal sector, and a subsidized one, which draws on those contributions and general revenue to cover the unwaged and those in the informal sector. There are well over a hundred for-profit insurers, complicating both choice and the provision of services.[135] The state says the system has 63,000 hospital beds and 5,300 for intensive care.[136] As of 2017, there were two doctors per thousand people.[137]

As is the norm with neoliberalism, what began with a supposed foundation in consumer sovereignty quickly became a centralized system of cost controls that determined which treatments were available to which people. Decades on, preexisting problems remain or have intensified: long lines, long delays, denial of service, and high out-of-pocket costs. Diagnostic technology and specialist opinions are increasingly restricted, while time spent with general practitioners is cut down again and again by insurance firms. Frustrated citizens generate logjams in the courts as they sue for adequate treatment. In 2010, a court ordered the state to pay for more equitable care. Even the government declared the system's "inequities a 'social emergency' in order to implement changes to the financing of public health."[138]

Of the country's 968 public hospitals, 40 percent were deemed close to financial collapse in 2012, putting ten million patients at risk. Costs of vital medications spiral as incipient capitalist corruption and industry pressure to outlaw generic treatments see Colombians paying some of the highest prices imaginable for vital pharmaceuticals.[139] Progressives blame these disasters on the profit-centered nature of health,[140] neoliberals on labor.[141] Those pesky workers . . . By contrast, things are very streamlined for affluent patients in private care.[142]

It is obvious that what neoliberalism regards as "reform" in these countries and elsewhere functions as corporatization and that it has been an abject failure in serving the collective interest. As per the infantile report cards and "top five" lists beloved of the bourgeois and so-called social media alike, tables like the Global Health Security Index are beguiling—and betray the cost of excluding political-economic factors such as the vain idiocy/hypermasculinity of conservative hegemons and the destruction wrought over decades by neoliberal lapdogs.

Political-economic analysis discloses that our dominant systems of health care have proven inadequate in planning for, providing against, and dealing with the current crisis. They must change, but so must public policy in general, to elude the nexus of disadvantage, inequality, and illness. Ironically, as per the 1973 oil shocks, the 2020 syndemic is a chance for wholesale political transformation. It is a limit case, where neoliberalism has been found wanting and can be displaced.

As Franklin Delano Roosevelt (FDR) put it when he ushered in the New Deal, it is past time to bid farewell to those who "know only the rules of a generation of self-seekers."[143] Forty years later, they roared back into town. *Eighty* years later, they must be dispatched for good. From the United States, from the United Kingdom, from Latin America. From everywhere.

You have failed. Go away.

2

During the Crisis

As the syndemic gathered pace, discussions and protests emerged over several issues: when a given state of exception, a lockdown, should commence and cease (something Colombians have lived with for most of the last eighty years but which is new to residents of Eagle Rock and Islington);[1] how to decide between the binary choice of public health and economic health;[2] and what kinds of societies we might hope for and seek to shape in the next conjuncture.[3] There were also struggles over allocating medical devices and medicines, from protective equipment for health workers to treatments and vaccines.

As we have seen, much health policy has been driven by phantasmatic, individualistic models of informed consent, responsibility, and decision-making that derive from the abstract playgrounds that trade as analytic philosophy and neoclassical economics.[4] Those reactionary ideas about responsibility and costs and benefits have long been the dominant discourse of professional bioethics and neoliberal policy formation.[5] Against them, in a certain sense, we are returning to the urgent, complex debates that ensued at the peak of the HIV/AIDS crisis.[6] At that time, activists called for new forms of clinical trials to hasten a cure and ensure equitable treatment for all. International organizations lobbied for pricing that would not discriminate against poor individuals or regions. Conversely, many scientists and governments sought to maintain established protocols. Corporations opposed any loosening of proprietary ownership of treatment in order to ensure they benefited from the drugs they helped develop. Today, the WHO's Ad Hoc Expert Group on the Next Steps for Covid-19 Vaccine Evaluation favors ongoing clinical trials for two years after COVID vaccines have been widely distributed, thereby leaving control subjects taking placebos in vulnerable circumstances. This would mean that a basic standard of care that has passed scrutiny was denied to many people, which would run counter to established ethical precepts. Anyone who watched *The Last Ship* will have seen these issues take dramatic form.[7]

Such norms have been brought into question through broader human-rights discourse, social research, and engagement with nongovernment organizations. They draw on different ways of thinking that are about empirical knowledge, justice, and solidarity rather than projections from a presumed monadic sovereignty; hence today's increased interest in applying One Health's doctrines to the present crisis, combining environmental, animal, and human wellbeing and acknowledging the importance of the Global South versus asinine anthropomorphism and unconscious immunoprivilege.[8]

Progressive work must transcend models avowedly based on consumption and engage the collectivities that form the actual core of societies: religion, housing, education, race, gender, age, class, incarceration, migration, refugee and conflict status, sexuality, criminality, animal and plant life, and so on.[9] Caring for others is part of our "social nature," as a few economists are belatedly rediscovering. Welfare is not merely about balancing incentives to work with adjusting to business cycles. It is part of the very fabric of life and should be based not merely on imaginary ratiocinative calculators but actually exiting humanity.[10]

Testing neoliberalism through empirical information—you know, research—is crucial to undermining it, but neoliberal expertise, such as it is, has also been problematized by the populist antiscience of harebrained politicos; giving in to ignorant demagogues essentially means accepting the foundational, ceteris paribus, myths of neoclassical economists. But the year of the mask has truly displaced the veil of ignorance that has forged, stoked, and distorted public policy for decades. Irrational populism is one reaction to that legacy. We can do better through a clearheaded account of the COVID crisis.

Latin America

Some analysts predicted a less drastic Latin American encounter with the syndemic than was the case in Spain and Italy, for example. This was based on climate, average age, and the speed and reach of quarantine measures, such as shutting borders, businesses, and educational institutions.[11] But tens of millions of Latin Americans had died when smallpox arrived with European colonists, and fears soon mounted as to this latest impact. Neoliberalism left most of the region in poor condition to manage the syndemic, the exceptions being Cuba (a socialist state) and Uruguay (until recently a social-democratic one).[12] The *Lancet* correctly notes that the syndemic's high death rates in Latin America are due both to the peccadillos of populist presidents and to long-standing inequality and corruption.[13]

At the time of writing (January 2021), the Americas provide five of the world's top twelve countries in infection and mortality, with forty-three million confirmed cases out of a global total of ninety-six million and hundreds of thousands of deaths.[14,15] With less than a tenth of the world's population, the region accounted for a fifth of global contagion and a third of fatalities.[16] GDP has fallen by a historic 5.3 percent, beyond the collapses experienced during the Great War and the Depression. Twenty-nine million Latin Americans have endured poverty for the first time.[17]

Just as the crisis is exacerbated by complex historical relations that foster inequality, discrimination, and violence, media coverage of the conjuncture has been hamstrung by the absence of both autonomous public broadcasters and pervasive digital access.[18] The lack of such services has been especially notable in education, where the fantasy of interactive distance learning is impractical for the popular classes. August econometricians estimate that the average cost of the syndemic to school pupils globally is already a third of a year, with effects on economic output for the remainder of the century. Ninety-five percent of Latin America's 150 million school pupils were sequestered at home in 2020. The longer that face-to-face instruction remained interrupted, the greater the subsequent economic impact; more immediately, the loss of childcare afforded by public education hindered the capacity of households to keep or retain paid work, with a disproportionate impact on women. Wealthy families supported private education, hired tutors, and showed little interest in public schooling, which suffered as municipal, provincial, and national governmental revenues fell. Meanwhile, college enrollment, which had doubled across the region this century—the world's fastest expansion—saw a massive drop in matriculation.[19] The students I teach in Mexico City have experienced parents, grandparents, siblings, and selves fall ill. Many suffer from food insecurity.

Mexico and Colombia must also deal with chronic tropical diseases, malnutrition, and tuberculosis. In addition,

Colombia has a huge internal refugee population: millions driven from their regions of origin by paramilitary, state, mafia, and guerrilla violence suffer abominable living conditions and health care.[20] As well as being a card-carrying neoliberal subaltern intellectual of the kind described in chapter 1, Duque is associated with a deeply authoritarian and corrupt political formation under the sign of his mentor, ultrarightist ex-president, rentier-class propagandist, and paramilitary patron and pardoner Álvaro Uribe Vélez.

By mid-January 2021, the nation's fifty million residents had suffered almost two million COVID infections and more than fifty thousand deaths.[21] The state reacted in its customary draconian manner, closing borders even to citizens and permanent residents and shuttering the formal economy, though it did allocate additional money for the health-care system to cope with the crisis and reduce tariffs on medical imports.[22]

COVID-19 has shone a spotlight on differences between the middle and upper classes and the marginalized peasant, poor, Afro-Colombian, incarcerated, Indigenous, and working classes (groups that frequently overlap). When the syndemic hit, the results were predictable: the risk of dying was highest among those without private health insurance and from the lowest socioeconomic strata, notably Indigenous folks.[23] The narcos grew in strength, the criminalization of protest intensified, and politico-economic corruption adapted.[24]

The rate of contagion in the Amazon basin, which also affects Peru and Brazil, shows how sizeable the problem is when articulated to systemic, immense inequality. Jail overcrowding has created hotspots of contagion. Perhaps 7 percent of all syndemic infection across Colombia has been in one prison. Inmates trying to break out of squalid conditions have been gunned down.[25] Violent threats and aggression against health-care workers have proliferated, as in the region more generally.[26] There are surges in the overall crime rate.[27] And romantic stories of Indigenous people retreating to forests to blockade themselves from COVID[28] neglect the fact that these environmental defenders are slaughtered week after week by right-wing assassins working for shady, shadowy mining corporations.[29]

Reports proliferate of abusive men luxuriating in the additional power over female partners provided by lockdowns, insisting they not leave the house for fear of infection—or murdering them.[30] Bogotá's first out queer mayor implemented a supposedly safe system for the gender-segregated use of public space, *pico y género*, based on Colombia's number-plate system that limits car use and hence pollution. The license-plate method has operated by only permitting numbers ending in odd or even numbers to be driven on certain days. The COVID system allowed men out on odd-numbered days and women on even. It led to violence against trans people and sex workers.[31]

The country's sticky oligarchy is as powerful as ever: Congress sought to buy thousands of surgical masks to protect its members, at great cost; medical personnel in the Amazon were reduced to sending smartphone videos to news outlets, having been denied equivalent protection. And when physicians report data on infections and deaths that do not suit the national government, they are dismissed as little old rent seekers.[32]

In Mexico, the syndemic arrived with the country convulsed by a reconfiguration of hegemonic forces. López Obrador combines liberal traditions, reactionary nationalism, rhetorical antineoliberalism, an Indigenous/rural base, evangelical religiosity, destructive development, anti-intellectualism, ignorance, and antifeminism. This contradictory ideology has generated particular controversy among technocrats, intellectuals, and the third sector. Accused of continuing the worst of authoritarian populism through an archaic, naive relationship with *el pueblo* (the people), López Obrador is seen as an architect of polarization between rich and poor. For instance, his flagship development project, the Maya Train, which is planned to cross the Yucatán Peninsula and connect coastal resorts to archeological attractions, is opposed by environmentalists, the Zapatistas, small business, and oligarchs.[33]

When COVID struck, the government's incompetence saw the fewest tests conducted of anywhere in the region or the OECD.[34] The president claimed to endorse health-ministry guidelines but rarely followed them as he wandered around the country greeting crowds without wearing a mask while repeatedly announcing triumphs over the virus. Morning press conferences saw him showing off an amulet that allegedly protected him from COVID-19, courtesy of his pastor, as he told us that if we gave ourselves over to someone apparently named Jesus Christ, we'd all be saved from the syndemic.[35] He went on to share with us that "miren, lo del coronavirus, eso de que no se puede uno abrazar; hay que abrazarse, no pasa nada" (look, this coronavirus thing, the notion that you shouldn't hug someone; we can go on hugging and nothing will happen). Sadly, he later contracted the virus, just like his fellow populist deniers Trump, Bolsonaro, and Johnson.[36]

López Obrador matters not only because of his rhetorical status as president but because Mexico has a deeply centralized political system, despite being a federation. To the extent that state and municipal governments can work against his antics, they have closed public and private institutions unrelated to nutrition and health. But the general public has had freedom of movement, as opposed to the lockdowns imposed in Spain and Britain, for example. Half-baked efforts to keep people from congregating in parks are barely enforced.[37]

Meanwhile, over 1.7 million Mexicans have been infected, and at least 150,000 have died. Many epidemiologists postulate a much larger figure given the disparity between deaths in 2020 and historic averages—a leap of almost two hundred thousand additional fatalities.[38] In late October, when the official death toll was just below ninety thousand, officials acknowledged the real figure was minimally fifty thousand more.[39] Some suggested it could be as great as fifty times the official numbers.[40] This in a country with a population of 130 million.

It is estimated that about 70 percent of deaths are related to comorbidities, such as hypertension, obesity, and diabetes.[41] Those conditions have radically increased with neoliberalism's industrialization of food and subsequent changes in the labor market, 51 percent of which is informal.[42] Years of neglect have seen public hospitals become risks rather than safe houses. Appalling shortages of qualified medical personnel and basic as well as high-end technology have led to scores of unnecessary deaths. All this while the administration has cut expenditure on health.[43] Reactionary fiscal policies pursued during the syndemic have been sufficiently asinine to draw criticism even from the IMF, which could not but recognize the obvious need to pursue growth over balanced budgets, a tragically senseless *nostrum* of López Obrador.[44] The country has the lowest deficits in the region—and the worst prospects for economic recovery. This is in keeping with the shrinking economy that he has presided over from the time of his inauguration, thanks to brutal austerity measures.

López Obrador's policy during the syndemic of lending to small business rather than granting them money has proven disastrous. Lockdowns pauperized small businesspeople as well as those in the informal sector because of this policy. Hence restaurateurs protesting under the banner

Abrir o Morir (Open or Die).[45] Meanwhile, the environmental impact of his undying support for the extractive and construction sectors will only be known in the decades to come.

As the president looked on from a bland but fatal blend of scientific ignorance and religious superstition, data emerged correlating affluence with survival from the virus.[46] The popular classes are confronted with lack of effective government aid, famished families, risks from street life, hospitals bursting with patients, and crematoria and cemeteries jammed beyond any imaginable capacity. Vendors in the informal sector complain that they are repeatedly told to stay at home but not how to maintain their households.[47] The result? Our current health crisis could see 60 percent of people fall into poverty.[48]

Then there is the violence. When the syndemic hit, sizeable social-media groups formed that were dedicated to sacking supermarkets and inciting others to do the same.[49] Medical staff frequently commute in mufti to protect themselves from street assaults.[50] Unsurprisingly, narco cartels did not observe the nation's institutional lockdown.[51] And new records were set for assassinations, driven by narco rivalry, misogyny, and desperation.[52] For example, on June 17, 2020, 117 murders were recorded. The victims varied from capo wives to political targets, from children to cartel servants. Despite the dispatch of a hundred thousand Guardia Nacional members and the effect of COVID shutdowns, the year ended with over thirty-five thousand homicides.[53] The corollary daily homicide averages are thirty-eight in the United States and fewer than two in Britain[54]—about which one reads, shall we say, a wee bit more in the international bourgeois media.

On the nation's northern border with the United States, tens of thousands of asylum seekers have been brutally incarcerated by DC during the syndemic, with stories trickling out about infection. As per the López Obrador administration's relationship in general with Trump, there was minimal critique of these human-rights abuses from the Mexican side.[55] And as the virus shot through the nation, with acute shortages of protective equipment for medical personnel, factories went into overdrive to produce such materials—for the United States. That's export-oriented industrialization at work. How very efficient.[56]

The United States and United Kingdom

On June 27, 1969, *Life* magazine published "Faces of the American Dead in Vietnam: One Week's Toll." It featured the names and pictures of 242 Black, White, and Latino servicemen killed over the previous seven days.[57] The images "had an impact on American perceptions of the nature and cost of the war. It was personal—and devastating," said the *Military Times* fifty years on.[58] For many, it signaled a turning point.[59] In emulation of *Life*, the *New York Times* published the names of a thousand COVID victims on May 24, 2020.[60]

The link was not only iconographic, for both disasters disclosed chronic state incompetence. The federal government has been entirely ineffective in its response to the syndemic, apart from those career public servants who operate with relative autonomy from partisan terpsichores. Most Republican lawmakers have eschewed or opposed public-health necessities, while religious institutions and restaurants have sought legal redress against their closure.[61]

Rates of infection and death have been greatest among minority U.S. populations.[62] As of mid-December 2020, the mortality rate for Native Americans was higher than that of other racial groups: 133 per 100,000 versus 123.7 for African Americans, 90.4 Pacific Americans, 86.7 Latinx, 75.7 Whites, and 51.6 Asian Americans.[63] Dozens of studies confirm the high likelihood of infection among Black Americans.[64] Historic discrimination against low-income minorities has exposed them to poisonous air, toxic water, food insecurity, and overcrowded housing. Those effects of environmental racism correlate with comorbidities associated with syndemic mortality.[65] The prison population in the United States is also deeply racialized, and jails are systematically overcrowded, leading to appalling rates of infection—one in every five prisoners. In addition, millions of people are wrongly arrested, briefly imprisoned, found not guilty, and then released after having been exposed to COVID.[66] As a consequence of these tragic indices of inequality and hence vulnerability, overall life expectancy in the country is sliding back to where it was in 2003.[67]

The syndemic has been utterly catastrophic for jobs, beyond anything experienced since the war, and the luxury of working from home is largely restricted to high-income earners with fewer debts and more savings than the proletariat.[68] But not to worry. The syndemic saw the Federal Reserve quickly print a trillion dollars for the banks to play with—yet another gift of public money that could have gone to health care, education, and the environment.[69] Meanwhile, the number of homeless workers in the United States was expected to increase annually through 2023.[70]

Conversely, by the time markets closed on December 7, 2020, the nation's 651 billionaires had seen their combined wealth leap by more than a trillion dollars since the pandemic shutdown on March 18. A trillion. That dwarfs both public debt and the COVID stimulus programs provided to ordinary people.[71] Goldman Sachs's profits rose by $4.5 billion in the fourth quarter of 2020; that looked shoddy next to JPMorgan Chase "earning" $12.1 billion over the same period.[72] Amazon thoughtfully offered to assist with vaccine distribution as part of a desired expansion into digital health and pharmaceuticals—and obtaining personal and collective information about health.[73] It clearly needed to do so—in the first ten months of COVID, the company's stock price had risen by a mere 65 percent and profits by $14 billion, and Jeff Bezos's fortune had increased by $75.6 billion.[74] Something simply had to be done. Meanwhile, well-heeled fellow travelers in the antivaccination and COVID-denial movements were hypocritically successful in obtaining U.S. government-backed relief loans during the syndemic: the Informed Consent Action Network, the Children's Health Defense, the Tenpenny Integrative Medical Center, the National Vaccine Information Center, and Mercola.com Health Resources.[75]

Should they require special kinds of prophylaxis, the super-wealthy could avail themselves of a "COVID-19 inspired shadow vessel concept called *Haven*," a buffer where visitors would undergo quarantine and testing, complete with onboard laboratory and hospital, prior to transferring to one's superyacht. While waiting, guests would have access to a submarine, helicopter, and diving decompression chamber.[76] As one does. Away from seagoing ventures, the rich piled into private jets for lengthy vacations and other leisure activities at almost "normal" levels under the laughable category of "business aviation," as opposed to "the Scheduled Airlines."[77]

Britain's handling of the disaster has been as tragicomical as its ideological imperial confrere. One in four children experienced food deprivation in the first six months, many going without food for a day or more.[78] And those already living in poverty fared worst when the syndemic hit.[79] The buffer against unpredictable catastrophes provided by savings was available only to a few. The poorest decile of families had more debts than assets, while the wealthiest 1 percent managed with five million pounds per adult on hand.[80] The middle class, largely able to work from home during the syndemic, generally maintained income, cut expenditure, and paid off credit cards—not something available to those in the secondary labor market and the outcome of not only the immediate crisis but foolish existing policies.[81] Housing indexed such disparities: lack of affordable dwellings with sufficient space and adequate infrastructure exacerbated the spread of COVID, while the rate of evictions stimulated homelessness.[82] The greatest impact of the syndemic was felt by people under thirty and with annual household incomes below £10,000. These were the most common victims of furloughs. Almost ten million people went into debt to survive. Conversely, over half of high-income earners unable to work because of COVID continued to receive their regular salaries.[83]

And as in the United States, infection and death are racialized, hitting Black and South Asian Britons the hardest,[84] though the way in which minoritization occurs in the United Kingdom means that the biggest migrant groups working there (Poles, Chinese, Brazilians, and Colombians) rarely appear as such in official statistics. Many Latin Americans in Britain lack papers and are probably reluctant to enter the public-health system.[85] Racism also imperils those working in dangerous circumstances within the middle class—most British hospital doctors who have died from COVID are minorities.[86]

Attempts to test people and trace the carriage of infection across the United Kingdom have been a fiasco, with the relevant science ignored and grotesquely inefficient private companies hired to do the work of public service. All too often, ill people were told to travel hundreds of miles to be tested and required to stand in line for hours. Despite there being forty-four NHS virology laboratories and numerous universities ready to play their part, the existing system was sidelined in favor of for-profit firms contracted with billions in taxpayers' funds. Those corporate facilities were swamped. Once again, neoliberal promises were not met. The government blamed subsequent delays on the citizenry.[87] And in calling on industry to produce ventilators on an emergency basis, it forgot that manufacturing had been destroyed by successive administrations. In short, "coronavirus has not ruined the UK; it has exposed the systemic ruin already there."[88]

Libertarianism and Conspiracy

Then there is the issue of Tweedledum and Tweedledee—libertarian and conspiratorial lies and folly that borrow and distort ideas and norms from the New Left to the postmodern, from social movements to identity politics.

Typical antinomies divided the libertarian part. On one side was a predicted return to a supposedly latent savagery lurking within us all, initially indexed in overly vigorous supermarket contests for sanitary masks, toilet paper, and packaged food. Survivalists await the second coming of *The Lord of the Flies*,[89] with guns, ammunition, and ideology at the ready in well-stocked shelters.[90] When Trump's acolytes attempted to censor scientists fighting both the climate crisis and this virus, many of us pictured billionaires equipping their bunkers with materials "liberated" from public storage.[91] The brutal violence at the heart of libertarian and conspiracy theories alike is obsessed with apparent infringements on individual autonomy while failing to address inequality, militarism, religion, race, gender, and sexuality. Little wonder that the *Collins English Dictionary* heard those hysterical outbursts and declared *lockdown* its Word of the Year for 2020, ahead of *coronavirus*, *BLM*, *furlough*, *self-isolate*, and *distancing*.[92]

On the other side lay a touchingly Panglossian celebration, a supposed renewal of civil society, allegedly evident from Mediterranean and Manhattan terrace- and stoop-dwellers serenading health professionals and their derring-do; citizens collecting food for those in need; and folks finding innovative ways to make love not war, teach their children well, and take exercise.[93] It's the putative equivalent of 1940s liberators or the spirit of the blitz—in fact, a horrendous moment of British murder, sexual assault, and nonviolent criminality[94]—but not to worry, chaps.

Then there are the conspiracies. My local holistic health-store proprietor in La Condesa says the Illuminati, Microsoft, and 5G towers are spreading COVID. In San Luis Potosí, folks believe the virus was created by the government and is sprayed onto the city each night from the air.[95] Various theories attribute the syndemic to a bioweapon unleashed by Beijing, Judaism, or Islam or a grand plan for surveillance via quantum-dot microchip spyware injected into gullible people hoping for inoculation. Swab tests are said to be designed to damage the barrier between blood and brain.[96] Colombia and Mexico have seen nurses and doctors assaulted as they leave work because bereaved relatives believe their loved ones died by design. This is quite a typical reaction worldwide during this, as other, public-health crises. Medical personnel are targets of rage.[97] The actual number of people subscribing to such conspiracy theories is subject to considerable debate.[98] That said, they have an important lineage, nowhere more powerfully than in the United States.

Fifty-odd years ago, the lapsed leftist Richard Hofstadter published his best seller, *The Paranoid Style in American Politics*.[99] Even then, in that mythical past of political bipartisanship, Hofstadter noted that Congress and elections seemed to be designed for "angry minds."[100] He used the word *paranoid* because it captured the "heated exaggeration, suspiciousness, and conspiratorial fantasy" that characterized the expression of this anger.[101] Hofstadter was suggesting not that these people were clinically ill but that they had the propensity to state unfounded and brutal ideas and then seek to put them into practice. The point was really about rhetoric—hence the word *style*. He discerned a repetitive tendency in the debating content and tactic of our speechmaking that sought to expose internal and external conspiracies against the "real" America. The enemy might be Catholic, Black, Jewish, secular, Russian, Marxist, or Masonic, and it might strike in the eighteenth, nineteenth, or twentieth centuries. Its identity changed—but the threat was always there, lurking, poised to destabilize republican virtues.

The persistence of ethnic and religious transformations in the population, and fear of cosmopolitanism, has fueled such fantasies across the ages, as more and more people appear on the horizon who look, sound, or genuflect differently. Paranoid politicians are afflicted with a terror of the past, present, and future, derived from such encounters with change and newness and the interplay of a death dance, with reality and fantasy intertwined.

Beyond the specific history of the United States, like many myths, conspiracy theories reference class, racial, and sexual struggles; the complicity of government and business in unequal life chances and experiences; and the common desire, shared by religion, science, and everyday talk, to explain the mysterious and the dangerous. A perfectly legitimate popular concern about big government and big business helps stoke imaginary conspiracies that metaphorize material concerns. Richard Hoggart records 1950s White working-class English suspicions that the new object called tinned pineapple was actually "flavoured turnip" (referencing long-standing European beliefs associating "turnip blood" with spineless behavior).[102] Patricia Turner's 1990s study of rumor in African American culture identifies contemporary beliefs that work through such tensions: the Klan is thought to own a national fast-food franchise, a malt-liquor company, and a soft-drink firm that sterilize Black men through additives. Whites and Blacks across the twentieth century ran a "Topsy/Eva" legend in which a Black or White preadolescent boy was castrated by White or Black men in a public toilet, respectively.[103]

Popular disillusion with technocracy, the electoral process, bureaucracy, diplomacy, the law, and other forms of state activity and cultural or intellectual expertise is neither new nor absurd. Nor is the attempt by demagogues to take advantage of the fact through antistatist appeals to those who feel disenfranchised. These lures are typically couched in opposition to politics by people posing as outsiders who are actually insiders or wish to become so.[104] But wholesale disaffection with the very nature of democracy and its checks and balances, to the point of deriding houses of review, the judiciary, policy analysis, scholarly knowledge, public service, and the press corps, as similarly tarnished with special pleading, corruption, and incompetence, is newly and devastatingly au courant. To understand these tales, we must listen to them in accordance with the notion of charity expounded by Donald Davidson—that to comprehend others, we must tie our own propositions and actions to theirs.[105] To write off conspiracy theories as products of "false consciousness"[106] is as unwise as to celebrate them as resistive. The point is to understand the urges that they reference and reorient them towards a political-economic redress.

The only popularly trusted state figures in the United States are the military and populist politicians. They are seen to have direct lines to the consciousness of the citizenry, whose drives and dislikes are to be trusted, always and everywhere. Checks and balances are deemed to be as ludicrous as elections—what matters is the spirit-in-dwelling of the nation, as magically incarnated in charismatic leaders and their irrefutable, incomparable organic connection to ordinary life, be they little-Englander Brexiteers, QAnon millionaires and workers, or acolytic Colombian and Mexican evangelicals obeying U.S. pastors. Regardless of these entities' actual links to privilege, power, wealth, or religion, they appear to be outsiders—antipoliticians who are admired because of what they oppose and because they have putatively emerged from beyond the conventional norms of electoral and administrative organization.[107] It is as if the triumph of liberal-capitalist democracy since the war, decolonization, and the decline of state socialism had masked an instability at the very heart of seemingly established constitutional arrangements.

Terror in the face of governmental surveillance is a core part of conspiracy theories, with epidemiological needs for knowledge of health and conduct deemed a threat to liberty. Against such Tweedledum and Tweedledee fantasies, we must recognize that state knowledge of the people has been a central strut of modernity since it began, making populations secure and productive as much as controlling them:

> An important problem for [French] towns in the eighteenth century was allowing for surveillance, since the suppression of city walls made necessary by economic development meant that one could no longer close towns in the evening or closely supervise daily comings and goings, so that the insecurity of the towns was increased by the influx of the floating population of beggars, vagrants, delinquents, criminals, thieves, murderers, and so on, who might come, as everyone knows, from the country. . . . In other words, it was a matter of organizing circulation, eliminating its dangerous elements, making a division between

good and bad circulation, and maximizing the good circulation by diminishing the bad.[108]

With the expansion of authority into the everyday, into all corners of life, the quid pro quo for the security afforded by governments is that our lives have become knowable. The equivalent expansion of *corporations* into the everyday, into all corners of life, has as its quid pro quo for the provision of goods and services by companies that they, too, know more and more about people: a core aspect of contemporary capitalist marketing *to* us and selling knowledge *about* us to others. Careful critics of surveillance who value privacy are torn between endorsing the need for knowledge of COVID's who-what-when-where-how questions and fearing additional corporate and governmental knowledge of everyday life that will not end with control of the virus.[109]

It is certainly true that the syndemic has both unleashed and legitimized racial and other human-rights abuses by states operating in the name of the greater good.[110] It is also true that "genomic surveillance" is vital as the virus mutates and that enforced lockdowns are effective against viruses and ultimately less corrosive for the economy than the disease itself. This was evident in China's dramatic return to growth following its shuttering of doors, because COVID had been effectively quarantined.[111]

The fact that conspiracy theories metaphorize real and pressing issues does not make them true. And just as protest and the use of spectacle pioneered by the left in the 1960s were corporatized over time, so they have been taken over by reactionary social movements. When I was young, the left had full ownership of conspiracy theories. Now it's the right, in all the countries I looked at for this volume, from my local storeowner to yanqui climate-change skeptics, evangelical true believers, and Brexit advocates. Their positions need to be heard, interpreted, and contested.

Alternatives

There are uplifting examples of grassroots reactions during lockdowns. Many people in quarantine or hospital celebrated the workers who cared for them. Supermarket employees were deemed essential; janitors essential; teachers essential. Clear skies treated *Chilang@s* (residents of Mexico City) to fresh air. Londoners and New Yorkers weren't subjected to soot on their windowsills or the unwanted feel of lank, putrid hair. The sweet sounds of birds singing were no longer interrupted by honking horns. Seismic activity around the planet diminished. While people paused their pursuit of unnecessary consumption, tourism, and waste, waterways cleansed themselves.[112]

And consider the Colombian dancers and roommates Carolina Caballero and Ana Milena Navarro Busaid. They continued performing over the first two months of being shut in. What began as a challenge became a systematic exercise, encouraging new dances; advancing reflections on the relationships between people, spaces, and objects; improvising with what was at hand; and reinventing relationships with the public. That involved the two performers confined in one house carrying out a daily exercise of experimental creativity. Each day, furniture was removed from the chosen room. The collaboration began with the choice of a reference for the creation to come: a fragment of a recognized piece, one or two objects, a place in their home, and musical or movement genre—from Pina Bausch to J. Balvin, Akram Khan to M. C. Hammer. Having made those decisions, a collaborative exercise saw movements chosen as starting points for improvisation. After rehearsal and practice, decisions were made about costumes, lighting, and recording devices. A collaborative video editing exercise was taped, edited, and circulated on social networks. Comments in response provided ideas for future creations.[113]

Our dominant systems of health care have proved inadequate in planning for, providing against, and dealing with the current crisis. They must change, but so must public policy in general, to ensure we elude the awkward nexus of inequality and illness. Ironically, as per the 1973 oil shocks, the 2020 syndemic is a chance for wholesale political transformation. It is a limit case where neoliberalism can be found wanting and displaced by the solidarity and inventiveness shown by these artists.

3
After(?) the Crisis

I don't envisage a quick and conclusive end to the syndemic—rather, I see a series of maneuvers by corporations, states, and populations in response to the disease and its socioeconomic effects. Such a patchwork narrative is not dissimilar to the oil story after 1973, when massive shocks eventually led to enduring change because the moment was seized by ideologues of neoliberalism—who had been beating the drum for some time. Now is the moment for their opponents to unite and undermine forever the dangerous but efficacious fictions that have hindered serious policy formation and implementation for two generations. That starts with an appreciation of citizenship.

The last two hundred years of modernity have produced three zones of citizenship, with partially overlapping but also distinct historicities: the political (the right to reside and vote), the economic (the right to work and prosper), and the cultural (the right to know and speak). They correspond to the French revolutionary cry "Liberté, égalité, fraternité" (Liberty, equality, solidarity) and the Argentine left's "Ser ciudadano, tener trabajo, y ser alfabetizado" (Citizenship, employment, and literacy).[1] The first category concerns political rights; the second, material interests; and the third, cultural representation.[2]

Political citizenship gives the right to vote, to be represented in government, and to enjoy physical security in return for ceding a monopoly on legitimate violence to the state (although the United States is contradictory about this issue because of the putative constitutional right to bear arms). Despite its focus on the nation and the state, the founding assumption of political citizenship is that personal freedom is both the wellspring of good government *and* the source of its authority over individuals. As developed through and against capitalism, slavery, colonialism, and liberalism, political citizenship has expanded its reach and definition. Although spread unevenly across space and time, the model is critical to every sovereign state. For its part, economic citizenship flipped from being oriented toward equality and instead became a selfish invocation of bourgeois individualism, part of neoliberalism's call to do good by doing well for oneself and the notion that corporations and capitalists are models for government. Cultural citizenship has been crucial in stressing that societies are mostly hybrids, as a consequence of colonialism and immigration, and that while everyone deserves equal treatment, particular needs and rights apply to Indigenous, disabled, and other structurally disadvantaged groups.

Citizenly reactions against neoliberal and populist fallacies proliferate today, such as Cate Blanchett insisting that the state "is not the same as business" because it should "regulate and guide the increasingly complex social landscape" as "part of our duty to each other."[3] But the project of citizenship is incomplete: "We all too easily take a non-sectarian civil life for granted, forgetting that in a proselytising religious culture it stands as an exceptional accomplishment. In fact the separation of spiritual discipline from secular government and conscience from law was never complete. It remains our own unfinished business, a contest unresolved since early modern times."[4]

What to do? Three partially overlapping yet different theories of public policy present themselves as counters to neoliberalism. They are implicit as well as explicit. Each one has something to offer, both analytically and practically.

The first theory concerns supranational government. The dream of liberal internationalists since the post–World War I invention of the League of Nations, it is incarnated today in the United Nations (U.N.) and has two elements.[5] One is a utopic faith in the possibility of transcending narrow national interests in favor of the general good of humanity. This goal has proven elusive because the anarchy of international relations is encouraged by economics, religion, and ethnicity. The U.N. is an avowed failure at keeping any kind of peace, and the disorder of world politics is intense.[6] The second aspect of supranationalism is more technical and has seen greater success. U.N. bodies such as the Food and Agriculture Organization and the WHO are occasionally branded as political (the latter most spectacularly during the current crisis) but have largely become spaces for the application of technocratic rationality. This less utopic faith in a disinterested expertise that can triumph through the power of objective evidence animating raison d'état remains powerful.[7]

The second theory of public policy views it as subject to competing interests, which determine its outcomes. Parliamentary democracies are supposedly open to numerous loud and cogent voices articulated to material interests and voting blocs. So the entrée of the extractive industries is clear when lobby groups, think tanks, political donations, and unscientific denial overrun technical expertise.[8]

The third theory of public policy holds that the state is inherently undemocratic and hopelessly compromised by interest groups, but activists can force citizens to watch, listen, and learn through spectacle—the fabled nonviolent direct action. This theory assumes that sovereignty resides in righteous indignation and universal values that transcend government and represent the popular will in an unmediated way via civil society.[9] Theirs is the authentic assembly, not the U.N. Once the province of new social movements, such as feminism and environmentalism, this terrain has been repossessed by Tweedledum and Tweedledee.

When we ponder the use of direct action and spectacle, it's easy to fall into either a critical camp or a celebratory one. The critical camp would say that rationality must be appealed to and competition for emotion will ultimately fail. Why? The silent majority doesn't like the avant-garde; marketing outspends art; such occasions preach to a light-skinned, middle-class choir; media coverage is slender; and crucial decisions are made in golf carts, not galleries. Many people experience activists as militant and eccentric, which foregrounds their otherness in such caricatures as tree-hugging hippies, ecoterrorists, antigrowth evangelists, economic ignoramuses, middle-class layabouts, vapid vegans, or romantic dreamers. While that otherness may be a core part of activist identities (behaving oddly in public, grabbing attention, securing column inches), its self-fulfilling politics severely limits the ability to communicate effectively across a range of constituencies.[10]

We have seen how their greatest successes have been, ironically, modeling irresponsible, childish conduct to libertarians and conspiracy theorists. And that "other" activism, of the right, has proven itself tied to violence in ways that are similarly linked to critiques of technical expertise and a passion for dressing up, marching, charging, and shouting.

For students of history and those in the Global South, it was little short of risible to be told by yanqui journalists and pundits, during and after the White right's temporary takeover of the U.S. Capitol in January 2021, that these events could only be understood—and shamefully so—by likening the country to a "banana republic." That forgot the role of the United States in exploiting the resources and dominating the politics of Latin American countries (which birthed the fruitarian adjective). We were treated to reporters on-site and commentators on Webex referring to the events as akin to being in Bogotá, Iraq, or other "trouble spots."[11] But for the left, conscious of these offensive, self-serving liberal shibboleths, the way that conspiracy-theory terrorists had used the politics of spectacle produced uncomfortable echoes of the popular resistance to tradition and reverence we have held dear.

Six decades ago, Tom Lehrer sang of how the left clung onto culture in the face of defeat. Looking back to the Spanish Civil War and the Lincoln Brigade's part in the struggle against fascism, he drolly noted, "He may have won all the battles," but "we had all the good songs," troping "Venga Jaleo."[12] That became even more relevant with the stress on cultural politics that came with the *soixante-huitards* and *les événements* of the 1960s, antiglobalization protests on the cusp of the millennium, and Occupy a decade ago. Today, the angry populist right chants, dresses outrageously, cocks a snook at authority, and opposes globalization and representative politics. The tools of resistance have been seized and used against the disempowered left by a disempowered right that is unknowingly articulated to corporate interests.

So do fine words and peaceful public protest have a place in helping transcend the current disaster?

On the occasion of his first inauguration, during the Depression, FDR coined a famous phrase: "The only thing we have to fear is [pause] fear itself."[13] Nice slogan. But such hortatory rhetoric can be worthless as a response to illness and conflict if it urges us to act individually. Whether through religious fervor or individualistic arrogance, that's just—well, stupid. For example, the second-century Roman emperor Marcus Aurelius was renowned for his stoicism. He helped shape an entire philosophical movement dedicated to it and provided this famous maxim: "Pain is neither intolerable nor everlasting, if thou bearest in mind that it has its limits, and if thou addest nothing to it in imagination."[14] Many of his fellow Stoics died of the plague while propounding the virtue of just such a stiff upper lip, thereby exposing them and their followers to intolerable risk. And in *Paradise Lost*, Milton toed the line, telling us that

> The mind is its own place, and in itself
> Can make a heaven of hell, a hell of heaven.[15]

Again, that rhetoric works well for those enamored of the brutal fantasies of religious zealotry who look to imagine their way out of peril or rational calculators who care about no one and nothing beyond themselves. It is laughable, pitiful—entirely inadequate—when faced with dangers that transcend collective superstition and individual ken. That's what happens when you must confront a shared danger: bombs, guns, men. Viruses.

FDR's 1933 paean against fear resonates most powerfully when it is read not as asinine bourgeois bravery but as a call to solidarity, to togetherness. And let's recall something else from his speech. It had more to say than its famous, overly stoic slogan suggests, for Roosevelt also emphasized the necessity of eschewing the "evils of the old order."[16] He was referring to selfish speculative capitalism, insisting that in its place there was a compelling need for "social values more noble than mere monetary profit" and for the U.S. government to act as a "good neighbor" throughout the region.[17]

I often turn to his words and to the memorable speech Bobby Kennedy gave on the campus of the University of Kansas during his brilliant, charismatic, but above all caring 1968 campaign for the presidency. Kennedy spoke that day of an "unselfish spirit that exists in the United States of America." He queried a definition of gross national product that "counts air pollution and cigarette advertising, and ambulances to clear our highways of carnage. It counts special locks for our doors and the jails for the people who break them. It counts the destruction of the redwood and the loss of our natural wonder in chaotic sprawl. It counts napalm and counts nuclear warheads and armored cars for the police" while excluding "the health of our children, the quality of their education or the joy of their play . . . the beauty of our poetry or the strength of our marriages, the intelligence of our public debate or the integrity of our public officials. It measures neither our wit nor our courage, neither our wisdom nor our learning, neither our compassion nor our devotion to our country, it measures everything in short, except that which makes life worthwhile."[18]

Inspired by such thinking, hundreds of thousands of Colombians, from across terrain, class, age, and race, decided in late 2019 that they had had enough of failed neoliberal economics and authoritarian policing—of money redistributed upward, the targeted killing of social leaders, ecological devastation, willful misconduct of the peace process, and the usual litany of oligarchic and oligopolistic self-satisfaction and parthenogenesis. They took to the streets against this persistent violence knowing that some of their number would suffer further brutality as a consequence.[19] Such activism has continued in the current conjuncture, along with efforts to protect the aforementioned environmental defenders and ensure their attackers do not operate with their customary impunity—a year later, students and workers across the country joined in protests that called for a basic wage for all, aid to small enterprises, and improved health care.[20] In a country laden with violence, with state brutality always at the ready, the courage of such actions cannot be overestimated—protesting peacefully in public is a real risk. It brought national and world attention to these issues, before and during the syndemic. Such peaceable bravery is a much-needed reminder of the right way to use spectacle politically.

We're already being told that even though we must rely on the state in the lonely hour of the last instance—which is assuredly this hour, this day, this month, this year—the future will see us pay financially and socially for the necessities of the present crisis; that we must go back to the economy as it was prior to COVID-19. The neoliberal newspaper the *Economist*, marked by its commitment not only to capitalism but also to democracy, science, environmentalism, and gender and racial equality (of "opportunity"), warned against any utopia forged from the rational use of government to provide a better life. It did so via an already-notorious cover story: "After the Disease, the Debt."[21]

Does that mean a return to austerity for the poor and the middle class and business as usual for the wealthy, be they beneficiaries of the military-industrial complex or other captains of casino capitalism?[22] A rerun of 2008 and neoliberalism's second inauguration?

It must not. The new lives that emerged from the horror of the Depression and the ashes of war should be our inspiration. Those lives were made possible not through nationalistic bluster or selfish consumption, but thanks to solidarity. The notorious flawed homology drawn again and again in the bourgeois media and by technocrats between household budgets and governmental ones is silly. As journalists, mandarins, and politicians warn that borrowing and expenditure will be rained on and reined in, they rely on decades of lies blinding ordinary people to the facts: that the United States and the United Kingdom have massive power over the price of money thanks to their central banks and can depend on financial forces to purchase their debt during crises at astoundingly low interest via loans lasting decades that can be repaid early when growth stimulates state revenues.[23] During the year of devastation, 255 million jobs were lost around the world, costing working people $3.7 trillion—and markets surged an average of 11 percent. Business as usual carried on for stockholders; it was disastrous for workers. The idea that debt must be repaid helps drive those market numbers and adds to woe for the women and young people who suffered most from disemployment.[24]

Despite neoliberalism's triumphs, elements of socialism for all remain—pesky, insistent monuments to sharing risk and cost in the collective interest. So education K–12 remains a (free) right. Railway termini, post offices, telephone exchanges, freeways, and electricity stations stand alongside public schools as physical and intellectual monuments to socialism. Unemployment and disability are compensated. Retirement and health are deemed shared responsibilities of the individual and the collective.

We can build on that imperfect, incomplete heritage of care to forge a brighter future. And health, which is both at the cutting edge of struggling with COVID-19 and the latest and most universal index of neoliberalism's failure, offers a way forward. As per the 1970s oil shocks, the 2020s provide a chance for wholesale political transformation now that neoliberalism has been found wanting; it can be displaced en route to 2100.

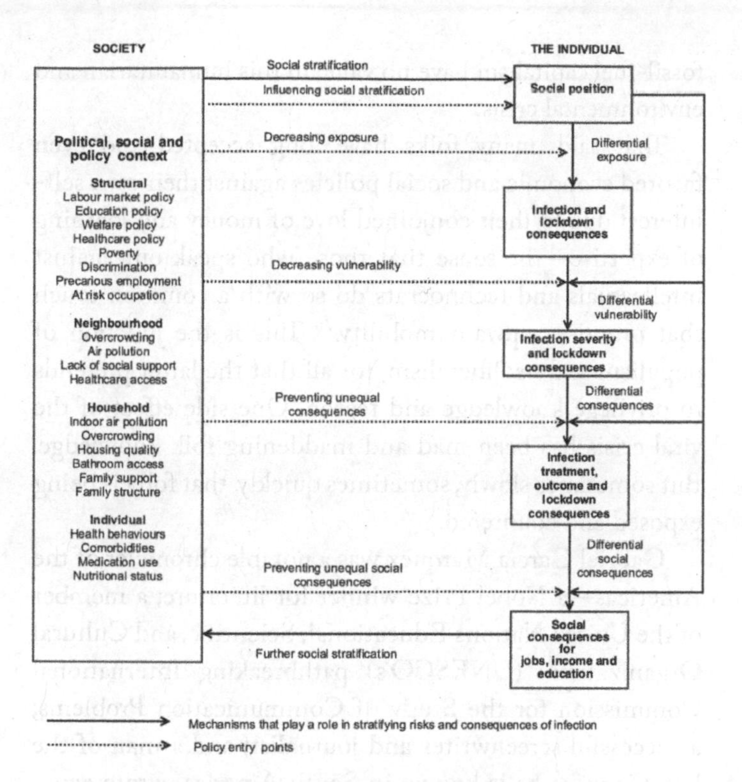

FIG. 1. *Source:* Whitehead, Barr, and Taylor-Robinson, "Covid-19," 2020.

Figure 1 depicts the ways in which industrial and finance capitalism and systematic inequality render a focus on individual desire as a poor basis for combating the syndemic. It suggests areas where interventions can be made.

We must now come to terms with the horrors of modernity, not only via technocrats seeking solutions to problems created by themselves or other technocrats but also via transparent decision-making that encourages public debate.[25] Why would we want moguls, meat eaters, and militarists to return to their destructive ways in a postsyndemic world? They are not role models in the realm of ecosystems and human health. The City of London, Wall Street, and fossil-fuel capitalism have no value in this humanitarian and environmental crisis.

That said, many folks have long accepted and even favored economic and social policies against their own self-interest due to their conjoined love of money and loathing of expertise—the sense that those who speak out against intellectuals and technocrats do so with a common touch that promises upward mobility.[26] This is the junction of populism and neoliberalism, for all that the latter pretends to privilege knowledge and reason. One side effect of the viral crisis has been mad and maddening folk knowledge. But sometimes slowly, sometimes quickly, that folly is being exposed and countered.

Gabriel García Márquez was a notable chronicler of the Americas—a Nobel Prize winner for literature; a member of the United Nations Educational, Scientific, and Cultural Organization's (UNESCO's) pathbreaking International Commission for the Study of Communication Problems; a successful screenwriter and journalist; and a man of the left. Gabo, as he is known in South America, wrote evocatively about a common dualism within the population of his native Colombia that spanned generosity and violence, warmth and hatred.[27] He described a powerful bifurcation coursing through the nation, the product of its particular pattern of invasion, dispossession, enslavement, and revolution. This resulted in a restless quest to identify the source of violence. Is it the nation, the right, the left, landowners, or the state?

At one point in *La mala hora* (*The Hour of Evil*), he decides, "Es todo el pueblo y no es nadie" (It's the whole town and it's nobody).[28] Gabo was referring to a place that was two countries in one—the ideal and the real—with all the associated paradoxes of a semiotic encounter between langue and parole, the rules of speech and its actual use, the abstract and the everyday. Although writing about Colombia, his great inspiration beyond his immediate environment was the southern United States.

Another Nobel laureate, William Faulkner, was García Márquez's model. And though the United States barred Gabo's entry for three decades—so fearful were we of his power to influence us—he never lost his appreciation for a great writer.[29] Why? Amid the rampant racism and developmentalism that Faulkner witnessed, in Gabo's words, that mellifluous, drunken, decadent novelist "refused to accept the possibility that mankind might come to an end."[30]

A similarly indomitable element of hope sustained García Márquez as a reader. As time passed, he feared that with it had diminished the very optimism that Faulkner insisted upon. While Gabo himself trusted that "life itself" could sustain us through solidarity, he saw with equal clarity that the loss of everything that Faulkner "feared is a straightforward scientific possibility."[31] Yet he never lost hope, believing that "it's not too late to build a utopia that would allow us to share an Earth on which no one would take decisions for other people, and where people on the margins would be given a fresh chance. A world in which solidarity could become a reality."[32]

Populist denunciations of expertise by López Obrador, Trump, Johnson, and their fellow charlatans around the globe look as hollow as they were once beguiling and must be displaced by an appreciation of material expertise that is based on solidarity rather than elitism. If we self-isolate and stay well, we liberate a hospital bed and respirator for someone in need. As our use of scarce materials declines, we pass spare supplies to the next population in need of care, who help others in an implicit antiviral social contract.[33] Such renewed solidarity, however compromised by religion, gender, borders, financial interests, and media bloviation, is crucial. If we can persuade the wider public that expenditure on the repressive state apparatus is wasteful, that academic knowledge can be valuable, that "faith" is obsessed with power and control, and that hegemonic masculinity has been bad for the vast majority of people, then life can get better.

If those truths about neoliberalism and populism are to percolate throughout society, we must explain how profound social inequality has become,[34] that this was not always the case, and that it need not remain so.[35] Furthermore, we'll need to show that the historic redirection of wealth upward has been achieved on the backs of ordinary people, to their disadvantage.

But we must not take the working class as the principal actor moving history forward. The multiplicity of social identities renders that form of thinking and call to action quite implausible. Instead, we must look for a socialism forged from the needs, pleasures, and labors of all progressive social movements in the struggle to overturn neoliberalism once and for all. In its place, we can install a vibrant new will to displace inequality with justice.

Many fields of thought emerged to counter the hegemony of neoliberalism during the syndemic. Scientists are being singled out as heroes.[36] They have shown what global cooperation can achieve when oleaginous profiteers, god-bothering true believers, and military blandishments are sidelined. Consider the rich collaborations that have permitted the emergence of protection and treatment against COVID-19: an international Coalition for Epidemic Preparedness Innovations; years of scholarly and commercial research into technologies capable of countering perilous genetic coding; Chinese scientists rapidly and openly identifying the virus and its RNA; adequate and immediate public funding in the Global North; experienced centers and personnel undertaking clinical trials; electronic gathering of data; sizeable numbers of volunteers; and medical-approval processes in pace with findings.[37]

That might seem as though everything went swimmingly. And indeed it has within the truly border-crossing community of scholarly science. But the success has also come because we have seen activism amongst these very scientists in the face of intransigent and incompetent politicians and ill-advised publics. For example, epidemiologists are not just creators of statistical projections that suggest rising and diminishing rates of infection.[38] They have spoken up and demanded a break with the past in the name of an all-important obligation of care—a collective duty to act in the service of all. And they are not alone.

Within environmental and labor studies, feminist economists bring the sensate body into social analysis along with other elements not generally assumed relevant by neoclassicists, because they commit the cardinal sin of transcending market pricing.[39] As part of an ongoing dispute with binary divisions between nature and culture, feminist theory has interrogated the notion of progress as productivist and accumulationist. Some strands posit an essential distinction between men and women that finds the former responsible for the theory and practice of environmental destruction and the latter conversely blessed and cursed with unshakeable connections to the Earth due to their enhanced experience of food gathering and preparation, reproduction, and caregiving.[40]

Ecological economists call for restraints on growth via governments limiting unbridled impacts on our future. They use varied forms of thought to comprehend and counter climate change. Carefully evaluating the technologies and materials that can support human populations and nature, they aim to avoid undue stress on all participants. An "Ecological Footprint" instrument measures environmental value rather than monetary exchange and prioritizes sustainable life over productivity and profit.[41]

And while we are all familiar with the discourse of costs and benefits as a common-or-garden orthodoxy of mainstream policy analysis that weighs up the positive and negative aspects of actions based on what they have produced in related or identical contexts, another form of thought is available: the precautionary principle. It holds that "our knowledge of the effects of our actions is always exceeded by our ignorance"[42] and lays the burden of proof of value and safety on those who would introduce potentially toxic substances or dangerous practices into the environment in circumstances where there is no scientific consensus about the consequences of such actions.[43]

No one has a monopoly on righteous conduct, from religious diehards to Marxist true believers, from anarchist narcissists to law-abiding citizens, from dipsomaniacal literary heavyweights to gun-toting survivalists. But most of us know the value of togetherness, of solidarity, of caring for one another and the world around us. That may come from the teachings of Jesus Christ, the science of immunology, the experience of team sports, survival in the emergency room, or life on the line. It is a lesson we might all heed—not only for our own good but for others, too.

Ultimately, control of the reins of government will be essential. In that regard, the three theories of public policy all have their uses: the technical possibilities of a world run on a rational basis through the application of farsighted knowledge, the skeptical capacity to counter sources of powerful malfeasance that distort the truth, and the magical self-anointment of spectacle-based activism. For dramatic change to happen, we must demonstrate to ordinary people that there is value in their experiences and opinions but also in formal knowledge (why airplanes can take off, how sound is recorded, the impact of energy use on the environment, or how immunology works).[44] In particular, we need to determine the right mix of perspectives in order to communicate and persuade, ensuring that states and corporations mitigate the syndemic in ways that articulate to wider transformations and displace neoliberalism.

I'm a socialist—by that, I mean someone in favor of collectivizing risk, opportunity, and safety, things that benefited my family in recovery from the Depression and the war. In the midst of those horrors, "Over the Rainbow" and all the beloved songs from *The Wizard of Oz* were penned by socialists.[45] These were no Stalinists overwhelmed by a banal socialist realism. They were clear-eyed optimists who hoped for a better world. They imagined socialized risk, where the core characters in their music would collaborate—not compete—to make a better life. Such intergenerational care has long been a centerpiece of African American and Indigenous economic and environmental thought.[46] Many of us seek the same things today, with good reason—albeit without my ideology.

Social psychology and neuropsychology indicate that the impact of ecological research on public opinion depends to a significant extent on its capacity to communicate across political lines, per *The Wizard of Oz*. People who do not regard themselves as directly affected by climate change may adopt proenvironmental values when stimulated to think beyond themselves and engage cross-generational impacts—to consider, albeit in an anthropocentric way, the lives of those yet to be.[47]

Collectivist approaches to our world can appeal to reactionary souls, provided they are not determinedly opposed to expertise and are genuinely conservative. Plato referred approvingly to the power of natural disasters to unmake "crafty devices."[48] When these "tools were destroyed," new inventions and a pacific society, based on restraint rather than excess, could emerge.[49] Francis Bacon recognized that we must "wait upon nature instead of vainly affecting to overrule her."[50] Edmund Burke acknowledged that all generations were "temporary possessors and life-renters" of the natural and social world.[51] People must maintain "chain and continuity" rather than act ephemerally as if they were "flies of a summer," thus ensuring "a partnership not only between those who are living, but between those who are living, those who are dead, and those who are to be born"[52] to sustain "the great primeval contract of eternal society."[53] Bentham, a thinker much beloved by neoliberals, asked of our duty of care to animals: "The question is not, Can they *reason?* nor, Can they *talk*? but, Can they *suffer*?"[54]

Therein lies a key, or at least a clue, to our postsyndemic future. Perhaps previously prevailing policy shibboleths and their attendant inequality and corruption will wash away as so many lackluster bottled messages, never to be seen again. We can but hope as we look dimly through a haze of horror and misinformation toward a different tomorrow.

4
The Charter

Charters give their signatories, readers, followers, and other interested parties clarity about a conjuncture's demands, hopes, and fears. Some are specific to particular populations, such as poets, feminists, or film directors, and others to particular causes, such as opposition to nuclear war or pollution. Some are addressed to quite limited readerships; others claim to speak universally.

The taste for such declarations crosses ideological divides. But they typically share one thing: from the Ten Commandments on, they are "ruptures, breaks, and challenges to the steady flow of politics, aesthetics, or history."[1] Or in this case, responses to a very, very *un*steady flow indeed. They are utopian codes, born of dissatisfaction, revolt, and organization.

The most notorious and efficacious charter is probably the 1848 *Manifesto of the Communist Party*.[2] It has been both a form of common sense, to be followed at all costs, and something to be abjured, always and everywhere. On the other side of politics lies the 1994 "Magna Carta for the Knowledge Age," which proposed that political-economic transformations have been eclipsed by technological ones: "The central event of the 20th century is the overthrow of matter. In technology, economics, and the politics of nations, wealth—in the form of physical resources—has been losing value and significance. The powers of mind are everywhere ascendant over the brute force of things."[3] Authored by neoliberals who had helped engineer the Reagan administration, its devaluing of labor and denial of the material world were lapped up by cybertarian fellow travelers. That discourse remains prevalent and has both drawn upon and "enriched" neoliberalism.

Charters generally display a monologic tendency. In Janet Lyon's words, "The manifesto declares a position; the manifesto refuses dialogue or discussion; the manifesto fosters antagonism and scorns conciliation. It is univocal, unilateral, single-minded. It conveys resolute oppositionality and indulges no tolerance for the faint hearted."[4]

Guilty. But can one be more inclusive and polyvocal than that suggests—or at least beaver away trying to be so?

This chapter contains the specifics of the COVID charter. It emphasizes the expansion and deepening of human rights as part of broader action against neoliberalism, drawing for background on such documents as the EU Charter of Fundamental Rights, the U.N. Charter, the African Charter of Human and Peoples' Rights, the ASEAN Charter, the American Convention on Human Rights, the Earth Charter, and others germane to the current crisis.

In terms of secular internationalism, the U.N. Charter has proven to be a foundational document since its promulgation seventy years ago, because it was designed to transcend the specifics of time and place in the interests of the greater general good.[5] The others referred to above take off from its precepts. For instance, the EU Charter guarantees a raft of rights, from freedom of expression to social security, in the name of solidarity and equality. As is the case with many such texts, it is meant to enshrine certain democratic rights that are deemed fundamental, *pace* what may be momentary popular majorities that oppose them, with courts of review the means of separating state powers.[6]

For the last quarter of a century, the U.N. has approached "human security" as much more than freedom "from violence and crime."[7] In 2012, it adopted a definition that incorporated "challenges to survival, livelihood and dignity" as obstacles to the desired goal that people should be able to "exercise choices safely and freely."[8] Those principles inform numerous statements emanating from international organizations and the scientific community in the year of the mask. The Council of Europe drew on them in its call for social rights during the syndemic, notably adequate working conditions, health care, and attention to the elderly.[9]

All those issues in turn touch on debates that began after the war with the discrediting of eugenics, the emergence of international human rights, and a discourse of informed consent to medical procedures, as embodied in the Nuremberg Code and the later Helsinki and Doha Declarations.[10] As is the fate of many endeavors in the field of human rights, these norms have never held the full force of law internationally or nationally but are of increasing importance as guidelines and sources of political argument. And they touch directly on health care as a universal entitlement.

Away from documents spawned and adopted by sovereign entities, political manifestos have also emerged from social movements. In the United States, the classic would be 1962's "Port Huron Statement." It is often taken as the point of emergence of the U.S. New Left. Drawing inspiration from secular internationalism, civil rights, pacifism, unionism, and a rejection of shrill anti-Marxism, it was crucial for blending the collective and individual aspects of social movements, where identity and politics merged. The New Left picked up on the magical mix of localism and universalism incarnate in the Black civil rights movement and the teachings of Martin Luther King Jr. and El-Hajj Malik El-Shabazz (Malcolm X).[11]

The lineaments of that heritage can be found in the extraordinary statements of principle emanating from the scientific community in the year of the mask. Scholarly voices dedicated to lost ideals of objectivity had had enough. Oppenheimer's notion of the "technically sweet" was soured by neoliberalism's overreach and populism's arrogance.[12] The syndemic saw political stances and manifestos adopted by august institutions of science that could no longer remain silent and complicit in the face of the ebullient maleficence of the United States and British governments, whose collective stupidity makes even Colombian neoliberal technocrats and Mexican evangelicals look vaguely competent. Vaguely.

For the first time in its 175-year history, *Scientific American* endorsed a U.S. presidential candidate in 2020.[13] *Nature*, always more socially engaged, did the same.[14] *EClinicalMedicine* wrote an open letter, "Dear Mr. President, You Can't Lie Your Way Out of This Pandemic!"[15] Manifestos about politics emerged from the *Lancet*,[16] the WHO[17]—for heaven's sake, even the hitherto almost stultifyingly lugubrious *New England Journal of Medicine*.[18] The *Oncologist* called COVID-19 a "Medical Pearl Harbor," so alarmed was it by the "Societal Fissures and Leadership Breaches" that the syndemic had revealed.[19] Many scientists rallied behind the *Lancet*'s calls to decolonize the disease and eminent public figures favored a people's vaccine.[20]

The *Lancet* redeployed insights from its Commission on Non-communicable Diseases to address the crisis. The commission has criticized dominant health and development agencies for focusing their inquiries and efforts on epidemiology to the exclusion of urbanization, lifestyle, wealth, and poverty.[21] The journal published a "Pledge for Planetary Health to Unite Health Professionals in the Anthropocene" to take account of the environment and social inequality[22] as part of an expansion of Hippocrates's principles in the *Epidemics*: "To help, or at least to do no harm."[23]

The WHO's "Solidarity Call to Action" seeks to realign responses to the syndemic as common goods, with research, treatments, vaccines, and technologies shared among all rather than privatized and rationed by and for wealthy nations and groups.[24] Its "Manifesto for a Healthy Recovery from COVID-19" links the need for a coordinated response to the virus with the necessity of reacting to longer-term, slower-moving environmental crises as well as future, dramatic syndemics, with a focus on healthy urban spaces, sustainable and secure food supplies, improved sanitation and water, and universal health care.[25] The Economic Commission for Latin America and the Caribbean (ECLAC) charter calls for a new social compact to make welfare truly inclusive in the context of the informal sector and the need for a more expansive and inclusive democracy that will eventually aid economic development.[26] The "Respectful Maternity Care Charter" derives from established protocols of human rights and WHO norms but also from a recognition that the syndemic has exposed and heightened "the damaging impact of inequities" and the need for universal guarantees and improvements to health care and specific maternity and newborn rights.[27]

The European Commission's "Manifesto for EU COVID-19 Research" emphasizes the necessity for fair international access to treatments and vaccines, a moratorium (albeit voluntary) on intellectual-property rights, and an eventual return on investment for big pharma.[28] UNICEF published a manifesto written by Italian teenagers on the postsyndemic future. It calls for solidarity; justice across generations; and education, the environment, and health-to-be public goods.[29] The COVID-19 Global Solidarity Coalition's manifesto takes health care as a fundamental right, along with protection of the vulnerable. It calls for a departure from corporate capitalism, in favor of cooperative economies.[30] "Degrowth: New Roots for the Economy," signed by a multitude of prominent intellectuals and organizations from dozens of nations, adopts the broadest of approaches, favoring an insistence on meeting basic needs for all, with health care as part of that transformation.[31] So universal guarantees of health, housing, and nutrition must take priority over economic growth. The group seeks a reversal of development norms and a shift toward degrowth, which will diminish the spread of diseases such as COVID-19.

Corporate chiefs are also charter fans. Nine heads of big pharma signed a declaration guaranteeing that their firms would produce anti-COVID vaccines to the highest scientific and ethical standards—while providing access in the manifesto to their stock-exchange addresses as they did so.[32] To be fair to them, marketing aside, this was clearly an undertaking contra Trump's call for vaccines regardless of clinical protocols. The *New England Journal of Medicine* called for a solid design and implementation of clinical trials against political efforts to hasten the approval of drugs without proven efficacy and safety.[33] The U.S. National Academies of Sciences, Engineering, and Medicine typically operate as technocratic gatekeepers, their estimable publications staying clear of political-economic realities and issues. But they produced a very unusual document at the height of U.S. vaccine nationalism that called for the allocation of such medicines based on transparent criteria and the general global good.[34]

Now is the time for a new socialist program that takes seriously the limit case we confront—a program that comes up with ideas from the past, present, and future to seize the moment, just as neoliberalism did so artfully, brutally, and disastrously fifty years ago. More than ten trillion dollars were spent by states to protect the social order from COVID-19 in 2020, tripling what was spent during the 2008 crisis, equaling the drop in GDP. That may "dramatically reset citizen's [*sic*] expectations about what governments can do for them."[35]

Marx explained that "social revolution . . . can not draw its poetry from the past, it can draw that only from the future. It cannot start upon its work before it has stricken off all superstition concerning the past."[36] To do so, we should begin with the exemplary *Care Manifesto*'s core insight: "Neoliberalism is uncaring by design."[37]

A future in which we tear off our masks does not mean narcissistic civil disobedience against public-health advice. It does not mean imagining the syndemic arose from cell phone towers, bankers, lizard people, or other scapegoats beloved of the populist Right. It means tearing down the structures and removing the plaster that have protected neoliberalism's principal clients—corporations and oligarchs—in the United States, Britain, Colombia, and Mexico for fifty years and more. It requires that we transcend "the hollow certainties of nationalism" in favor of "a transnational orientation of care towards the stranger."[38] It takes inspiration from the reply that a rightly bemused Jonas Falk gave Ed Murrow when asked, "Who owns the patent on this [poliomyelitis] vaccine?" Falk said, "Well, the people, I would say. There is no patent. Could you patent the sun?"[39]

So here goes.

The COVID Charter

1. Inequality within and between countries is the key to the devastation wrought by the syndemic.
2. A guaranteed income for all must be introduced, based on taxes of the superwealthy.

3. Failure to provide adequately funded socialized health care to all has proven disastrous, as per rising levels of infection and inequality.
4. Environmental irresponsibility and the industrial slaughter of animals have been as central as evolution to the spread of the disease.
5. The industrial production and trade in meat must end.
6. Collaboration and the work of government are fundamental to innovation and public welfare.
7. Health research undertaken for motives of profit versus inquiry and the public good does not ensure an equitable allocation of the resources that derive from its findings.
8. A new U.N. agency dedicated to scientific research should take over part of UNESCO's mandate, funded by a levy on the biggest pharmaceutical corporations and financing collaborative research by teams from the Global South and North.
9. Health insurers should be socialized.
10. Public campaigns to educate people in the principles of epidemiology must begin in early schooling.
11. The bourgeois media must promise to adjudicate accurately when lies are told about scientific consensus.
12. Politicians unschooled in the relevant areas should stop denouncing expertise.
13. The so-called social media must be regulated as are other communications companies by independent bodies that stand to one side of government but have statutory power.
14. Current and former imperial powers must accept immigrants from nations they invaded and occupied.
15. Reparations must be paid to victims of slavery and trafficking.
16. Indirect taxes should be levied on luxury goods and firms that sell legal but dangerous products.
17. Wealth taxes should preclude the inheritance of stock.

18. A levy should be imposed on the international trade in material and virtual currency.
19. Accountancy firms should be socialized under the control of statutory authorities at arm's length from states.
20. Military expenditure should be cut in half in all nations, with the resultant savings directed to health, education, and elder care.
21. Children should receive a trust fund at birth.
22. Education should be a right K through college.
23. Pay for those giving care to others should exceed all executive and administrative salaries.
24. Recovery programs must cut 30 percent of greenhouse emissions by 2025.
25. Green spaces must be expanded and the poles, forests, waterways, and jungles protected from the extractive sector.
26. Freeway systems must include designated areas for bicycles safely blocked off from vehicular traffic.
27. Housing should be socialized and made fit for everyone.
28. Disabled and elder care should be the responsibility of the state and governed by those affected.
29. There must be emancipation of nonviolent offenders.

Acknowledgments

Thanks are due to Kimberly Guinta and Micah Kleit for supporting this wee project and to their fellow workers for bringing it to completion.

I very much appreciate the unnamed reviewers of the original proposal for their suggestions and the encouragement of collaborators on related projects: André Dorce Ramos, John Edwards, Nancy Regina Gómez Arrieta, Helena Grehan, Felicitas Holzer, Petros Iosifidis, Isabel Cristina Ramírez Botero, Jorge Saavedra Utman, Anne Schwenkenbecher, Federico Guillermo Serrano López, Ana Rita Sequeira, and Enrique Uribe Jongbloed.

I have been sequestered in Mexico City during the pandemic—initially due to lockdowns, then as a consequence of my migration status. I wish to thank people near and far who have so kindly helped me throughout this period, from folks in coffee shops to such friends and colleagues as Akuavi Adonon, Pal Ahluwalia, Ece Algan, Peter Anderson, Jesús Arroyave, Claudia Arroyo Quiroz, Paulina Aroch Fugellie, Sarah Berry, Edward Buscombe, Jo Clifford, Richard Collins, Joselyne Contreras Cerda, Stuart Cunningham, Talitha Espiritu, Natalie Fenton, Des Freedman, Néstor García Canclini, Faye Ginsburg, Rodrigo Gómez García, Lalitha Gopalan, Michael Gordon-Smith, Bill Grantham, Brían Hanrahan, Steve Harney, Joke Hermes, Kevin Hewison,

Richard Higgott, James Jacobs, Louise Katz, Alisa Kennedy Jones, Noel King, Amalia Leguizamón, Justin Lewis, Emilienne Limón, Jo Littler, Janet Lyon, Scott MacKenzie, Ana Rosas Mantecón, Richard Maxwell, Benjamin Mayer Folkes, Vicki Mayer, John McMurria, Gabriela Méndez Cota, Acácia Mendonça Rios, Marta Milena Barrios, Caitlin Miller, Lainey Paloma Miller, Beatriz Miranda, Vijay Mishra, Daniela Inés Monje, Rob Nixon, Tom O'Regan, Rune Ottosen, Jack Qiu, Arvind Rajagopal, James Ramey, Wendy Raschke, Adriana Reygadas, Luis Reygadas Robles, Kristina Riegert, Garry Rodan, Andrew Ross, Horst Ruthrof, Luz María Sánchez Cardona, Tom Scanlon, Dan Schiller, Rita Shanahan, Paul Smith, Anamaria Tamayo Duque, Serge Tampalini, Susana Vargas Cervantes, Aimée Vega Montiel, Gary Wickham, ShinJoung Yeo, George Yúdice, and Audrey Yue.

Thanks also to three writers for their thoughts on pandemics as history and fiction. Here is Samuel Pepys's diary entry from January 16 and 17, 1666: "Home late at my letters, and so to bed—being mightily troubled at the news of the plague's being increased, and was much the saddest news that the plague hath brought me from the beginning of it, because of the lateness of the year, and the fear we may with reason have of its continuing with us the next summer."[1] Next to Daniel Defoe's fictionalized *Journal of the Plague Year*, which referred to "the last great visitation," as if all were behind us.[2] And finally and conversely, the last sentence of Albert Camus's *The Plague*: "The plague bacillus never dies or disappears for good . . . it can lie dormant for years and years in furniture and linen-chests . . . it bides its time in bedrooms, cellars, trunks, and bookshelves . . . perhaps the day would come when, for the bane and the enlightening of men, it would rouse up its rats again and send them forth to die in a happy city."[3]

Most of all, my thanks go to Caitlin and to Lainey Paloma. I always miss you when we are apart, but never as much as now.

Notes

Introduction: The Year of the Mask

1 Marx 1951, 12.
2 Althusser 1969, 99.
3 Gramsci 2000.
4 https://covid19.who.int/?gclid=CjwKCAiAkan9BRAqEiwAP9X6UZZsR332ikMzOFWBYKP56Lepi7u2GTpFeamVaHKD5FGRIefgZ2PBehoCBGQQAvD_BwE; WHO 2021.
5 Marx 1951, 12.
6 Gramsci 1971.
7 Foucault 1980, 1982; Wade 2020.
8 Polese, Williams, and Hordonic 2017.
9 Akiyama, Spaulding, and Rich 2020.
10 Harman et al. 2020; O'Donnell 2020; Dlamini 2020.
11 Orcutt et al. 2020; Tchekmedyian and Winton 2020.
12 Engels 1946, 6.
13 Engels 1946, 6.
14 Adorno 1975, 18.
15 Latour 2004, 1, 33.
16 Latour 1993.
17 Quoted in Watts 2020.
18 Virchow 2006.
19 Foucault 2003, 247.

20 Singer et al. 2017.
21 R. Horton 2020.
22 Kant 2011, 17.
23 Merton 1936.
24 Honigsbaum 2020.
25 World Economic Forum 2021.
26 García Canclini 2020.
27 Roy 2020.
28 Marx 1951, 13.
29 Sen 2009, 248.
30 Kevany and Carstensen 2020.
31 *France 24* 2020.
32 Kevany 2020.
33 Wallace 2016.
34 *Economist* 2020c.
35 UNEP and International Livestock Research Institute 2020.
36 Taylor, Latham, and Woolhouse 2001; Davis 2020, 14–16; Quammen 2012.
37 UNEP 2020, xiii.
38 Tollefson 2021.
39 *Economist* 2021b.
40 Pfizer 2020.
41 Pfizer 2020.
42 *Forbes Mexico* 2020.
43 Kollewe 2020.
44 https://www.sec.gov/Archives/edgar/data/78003/000122520820013318/xslF345X03/doc4.xml.
45 *Economist* 2020b.
46 YouTube 2010.
47 Quoted in Chappell 2020.
48 Quoted in Oltermann 2020.
49 Moderna 2020.
50 Grady 2020.
51 CDC 2021.

52 Campbell 2020; NIH 2021.
53 Adhanom Ghebreyesus 2020, 2021.
54 YouTube 2021.
55 Doucleff 2020; Grady 2020; Voysey et al. 2021; Polack et al. 2020.
56 Government of Canada / Gouvernement du Canada n.d.
57 OXFAM 2020; https://peoplesvaccine.org; https://www.gavi.org; Coalition for Epidemic Preparedness Innovations, Gavi, and WHO 2021; *Nature* 2021.
58 Guillot 2021.
59 Ledford 2021.
60 Adhanom Ghebreyesus 2021.
61 Independent Panel for Pandemic Preparedness and Response 2021.
62 Paltiel et al. 2021; *Nature* 2020b; Adhanom Ghebreyesus 2021.
63 WHO 2020a; Mahase 2020; Muik et al. 2021.
64 Boseley 2021; Cele et al. 2021.

Chapter 1: Before the Crisis

1 Economist Intelligence Unit, Nuclear Threat Initiative, and Johns Hopkins Bloomberg School of Public Health Center for Health Security 2019, 20–22.
2 Economist Intelligence Unit, Nuclear Threat Initiative, and Johns Hopkins Bloomberg School of Public Health Center for Health Security 2019, 20–22.
3 Biden 2021; https://covid19.who.int/?gclid=CjwKCAiAkan9BRAqEiwAP9X6UZZsR332ikMzOFWBYKP56Lepi7u2GTpFeamVaHKD5FGRIefgZ2PBehoCBGQQAvD_BwE.
4 Hobbes n.d., chapter xiii.
5 Foucault 2004, 245.
6 Foucault 1978, 143; 1991a, 92–95, 97; 1991b, 4.
7 Foucault 2003, 241.
8 Foucault 2003, 241.
9 Foucault 1991b, 277.

10 Dorling 2013.
11 Synnott 2002.
12 Polanyi 2001.
13 Fogel 1993, 312–313.
14 Arminen 2010.
15 Emmison 1983; Emmison and McHoul 1987.
16 Foucault 2008, 216.
17 Jordan, Tumpey, and Jester n.d.; Arnold 2018; Bristow 2012, 60.
18 Mitchell 2011.
19 Hall et al. 2013.
20 Said 1999.
21 Shepherd and Stone 2013.
22 Bourdieu 1998, 94.
23 Malpas 1992.
24 Lockie 2017.
25 Ross 1996.
26 Lyotard 1988, xi.
27 Baudrillard 1988.
28 Mirowski and Plehwe 2009.
29 Foucault 2008, 247.
30 Gorbachev 2009; Hall and Massey 2010.
31 Brown 2019, 12.
32 Friedman and Friedman 2002, viii.
33 Oreskes and Conway 2010; Funk and Rainie 2015; Readfearn 2015; Dorling 2014.
34 Mayer 2016; Nelson 2019.
35 https://www.atlasnetwork.org/partners.
36 Stone 2013; Lawrence et al. 2019.
37 Dunlap and Jacques 2013; Anshelm and Hultman 2014; Hart and Feldman 2014.
38 Lewandowsky et al. 2015; Maxwell and Miller 2016.
39 Hardin 1968 is the locus classicus.
40 Agamben 2009, 9–10.
41 Becker 1993 is the apotheosis of this Olympian worldview.

42 Quoted in Keay 1987, 9.
43 https://www.youtube.com/watch?v=FOx8q3eGq3g&ab_channel=jascowo.
44 Quoted in Venegas 2003.
45 Varoufakis 2020.
46 Foucault 2008, 253.
47 Jensen 2007.
48 Mazzucato 2015.
49 AEC 1954.
50 Marx 1987.
51 Eisenhower 1961.
52 Knight, Loayza, and Villanueva 199.
53 Desli and Gkoulgkoutsika 2020.
54 Peace Alliance 2015.
55 https://www.youtube.com/watch?v=KbWTl82ZL_k.
56 Also see Folbre 2010.
57 Harrington 1962.
58 Quiggin 2010.
59 Fitzgerald 1926.
60 Dow 1988.
61 Hemingway 2016, 9311.
62 *Economist* 2006.
63 Kraus, Côté, and Keltner 2010; White 2020.
64 Leal Filho et al. 2018.
65 Caiani and Guerra 2017; Boykoff and Yulsman 2013.
66 Barclay 2018; Marcos Recio, Vigil, and Zaldua 2017; House of Commons 2019; Renda 2018.
67 https://languages.oup.com/word-of-the-year/2016/.
68 Williams and Delli Carpini 2011; Allcott and Gentzkow 2017; Marcos 2016.
69 Mudde 2017; Mudde and Kaltwasser 2017; Muller 2016; Mounk 2018; Mouffe 2018.
70 Hopkin 2020; Chakrabortty 2020c.
71 Mazzucato 2020.

72 Dorling 2014.
73 Hopkin 2020.
74 Kruse 2015; Maxwell and Shields 2019.
75 Miller 2008; Reich 2020; Blanchflower and Oswald 2020; Case and Deaton 2020.
76 Miller 2008.
77 Burtless 2014.
78 Miller 2008.
79 Price and Edwards 2020.
80 White 2020.
81 Piketty 2018.
82 Hope and Limberg 2020.
83 Lonergan and Blyth 2020, 46–47.
84 Innes 2020.
85 Chakrabortty 2019, 2020a.
86 Joseph Rowntree Foundation 2021.
87 Cárdenas, Ocampo, and Thorp 2000.
88 Rodrik 2007, 20.
89 ECLAC 2019.
90 Offner 2019.
91 North and Clark 2018.
92 Marmot 2004.
93 *Lancet* 2020.
94 Allier-Montaño and Crenzel 2015.
95 McPherson 2016.
96 Transparency International 2017; Anti-corruption Resource Centre et al. 2013.
97 Hellinger 2015, 326; Piketty 2014, 327.
98 IMF 2019; EIU 2019.
99 OXFAM 2016, 5–6.
100 *BBC News Mundo* 2018.
101 *Animal Político* 2017.
102 Levy 2008.
103 Herrera de la Fuente 2016.

104 Fine and Durán Ortiz 2016, 14.
105 Butt et al. 2019.
106 Global Witness 2019.
107 Giraldo Durán and de Castillo 2018.
108 Frenk and Moon 2013.
109 Morgenthau, Thompson, and Clinton 2005; Carr 1964.
110 Shaw n.d.
111 Miller 2008.
112 Fugh-Berman 2005.
113 Healy et al. 2003; Moynihan 2004.
114 Moffatt and Elliott 2007, 19.
115 Busch et al. 2004.
116 Mirowski 2011.
117 Sismondo 2013.
118 Emanuel, Zhang, et al. 2020.
119 Chapin 2015.
120 Miller 2008.
121 Reich 2020.
122 Reich 2020.
123 Reich 2021.
124 Hall et al. 2015.
125 Quoted in Germain 2020, 360.
126 Le Fanu 2005; *Social Insurance and Allied Services* 1942.
127 Dorling 2013; Chatzidakis et al. 2020, 48.
128 Faculty of Intensive Care Medicine 2017.
129 *Lancet* 2020.
130 PAHO n.d.
131 World Bank n.d.-a, n.d.-b.
132 Flamand 2020.
133 Urquieta-Salomón and Villarreal 2016; Barraza-Lloréns et al. 2002; Arredondo and Nájera 2008.
134 Webster 2012a.
135 Webster 2012a, 2012b.
136 Torrado 2020.

137 CIA 2020.

138 Webster 2012a.

139 IFARMA and AIS 2009.

140 Guzmán Urrea 2016.

141 Giménez et al. 2019.

142 Guzmán Urrea 2016.

143 Roosevelt 1933. The complete speech can be heard at http://audio.theguardian.tv/sys-audio/Guardian/audio/2007/04/24/FDRfinal.mp3, and part of it can be seen at https://www.youtube.com/watch?v=amNpxQANkoM.

Chapter 2: During the Crisis

1 Owen 2020.

2 Maxwell and Miller 2020a.

3 Maxwell and Miller 2020b.

4 Baron 2006.

5 Emanuel, Persad, et al. 2020.

6 Treichler 1999; Nguyet Erni 1994.

7 WHO Ad Hoc Expert Group on the Next Steps for Covid-19 Vaccine Evaluation 2021; Dal-Ré, Orenstein, and Caplan 2021; *The Last Ship* aired on TNT from 2014 to 2018.

8 Häsler et al. 2014; Ahmad and Hui 2020; Olivarius 2020; One Health Initiative n.d.

9 Satomi et al. 2020; Caplan and Arp 2013; Ebrahim and Memish 2020; Tsai and Wilson 2020; Van Lacker and Parolin 2020; Bhala et al. 2020; Wenham, Smith, and Morgan 2020; Coker 2020; Wilkinson and Pickett 2020; Rangel, Daniels, and Phillips 2020; Peter 2020; Nott 2020; Griffin and Rivera Antara 2020.

10 Saez 2021.

11 Amariles et al. 2021.

12 Wallis and Zhuo 2020.

13 *Lancet* 2020.

14 J. Horton 2020; https://covid19.who.int/?gclid=CjwKCAiAkan9BRAqEiwAP9X6UZZsR332ikMzOFWBYKP56Lepi7u2GTpFeamVaHKD5FGRIefgZ2PBehoCBGQQAvD_BwE.

15 Of course, testing regimes vary wildly in their thoroughness, from the incoherent incompetence of the United Kingdom to the extraordinary completeness of Cuba.

16 McDonnell and Linthicum 2020.

17 Bárcena and Reed 2020.

18 Mueller and Taj 2020.

19 Schleicher 2020; *Economist* 2020a; Hershberg, Flinn-Palcic, and Kambhu 2020; Neidhöfer, Lustig, and Tommasi 2020.

20 Webster 2012b.

21 *El Tiempo* 2020; https://covid19.who.int/region/amro/country/co.

22 IMF 2020a.

23 Cifuentes et al. 2020.

24 Castro et al. 2020; Saldarriaga 2020.

25 Rangel, Daniels, and Phillips 2020.

26 Taylor 2020; Palos 2020.

27 *BBC News* 2020a.

28 Collyns et al. 2020.

29 Oquendo 2020.

30 Gearin and Knight 2020; Parkinson 2020.

31 Griffin and Rivera Antara 2020; https://twitter.com/hashtag/PicoYG%C3%A9nero?src=hashtag_click.

32 Alsema 2020.

33 Godoy 2020.

34 Fowler et al. 2020.

35 Kitroeff and Villegas 2020; https://www.youtube.com/watch?v=Hf6vI5uODYc&ab_channel=Ruptly.

36 Urrutia 2021.

37 Flamand 2020.

38 https://covid19.who.int/region/amro/country/mx.

39 Phillips 2020.

40 Fowler et al. 2020.
41 *Animal Político* 2020; Singer 2020.
42 *Sin Embargo* 2020.
43 Kitroeff and Villegas 2020; Christensen, Fischer, and Shultz 2020.
44 IMF 2020b.
45 Deutsche Welle 2021.
46 Webber 2021; Millán-Guerrero, Caballero-Hoyos, and Monárrez-Espino 2020.
47 Quintero Morales 2020; McDonnell and Linthicum 2020.
48 *Sin Embargo* 2020.
49 Camhaji 2020.
50 Agren 2020.
51 Balmori de la Miyar, Hoehn-Velasco, and Silverio-Murillo 2020.
52 Ferri 2020a and 2020b.
53 Grant 2020; Angel 2021.
54 FBI 2019; Office for National Statistics 2020.
55 Slack and Heyman 2020.
56 Sieff 2020.
57 Cosgrove 1969.
58 Wright 2019.
59 Maxwell and Miller 2020c.
60 *Guardian* 2019.
61 Kaplan 2020.
62 Carpenter 2020.
63 APM Research Lab 2021.
64 Sze et al. 2020.
65 Washington 2020; Cole and Foster 2001.
66 Jones 2020; Franco-Paredes et al. 2020; Reinhart and Chen 2020; Associated Press 2020.
67 Andrasfay and Goldman 2021.
68 Handwerker et al. 2020; *Economist* 2020c.
69 Reich 2020.
70 Flaming et al. 2021.
71 Americans for Tax Fairness and Institute for Policy Studies 2020.

72 *Economist* 2021c.
73 Luthi 2021.
74 Kinder, Stateler, and Du 2020; Kinder and Stateler 2020.
75 Cowley 2021.
76 Incat Crowther 2020.
77 WINGX 2021.
78 Bhattacharya and Shepherd 2020.
79 Joseph Rowntree Foundation 2021.
80 Advani, Bangham, and Leslie 2021.
81 Bank of England n.d.; StepChange 2020; Gardner, Gray, and Moser 2020.
82 Tinson and Clair 2020.
83 Office for National Statistics 2021.
84 Sze et al. 2020.
85 Miller 2018.
86 Chakrabortty 2020e.
87 Chakrabortty 2020b.
88 Chakrabortty 2020d.
89 Golding 1954.
90 AFP and Borbon 2020; Diss 2020.
91 Rupar 2020; Waters 2018; Johnson 2020.
92 https://www.collinsdictionary.com/woty.
93 Rusbridger 2020.
94 Overy 2020.
95 Palos 2020.
96 Sutton and Douglas 2020; Stein et al. 2021.
97 Sheridan, Masih, and Cabato 2020; Trejos-Herrera, Vinaccia, and Bahamón 2020; Ramasubba Reddy et al. 2019.
98 Sutton and Douglas 2020.
99 Hofstadter 1966.
100 Hofstadter 1966.
101 Hofstadter 1966.
102 Hoggart 2009, 140.
103 Turner 1993, 2–3, 73, 149–150, 227.

104 Ionescu and Gellner 1969; Canovan 1981; Taggart 2000; Panizza 2005.

105 Davidson 2004, 35.

106 Engels 1893.

107 Cherniavsky 2017; Curini 2018; De La Torre 2015; Kriesi and Pappas 2015; Moffitt 2016.

108 Foucault 2007, 54.

109 Daskal 2020.

110 Amnesty International 2020.

111 Cyranoski 2021; Correia, Luck, and Verner 2020; *Economist* 2021a.

112 Maxwell and Miller 2020a; Koren 2020.

113 Ramírez and Miller 2020.

Chapter 3: After(?) the Crisis

1 Martín-Barbero 2001, 9.

2 Rawls 1971, 61.

3 Blanchett 2020.

4 Saunders 1997, viii.

5 Laqua 2011.

6 Sjoberg 2013; Miller 1984; Bull 2012.

7 Cox and Jacobson 1974; Claude 1971.

8 Lindblom 1980; Hill 2012.

9 Graeber 2002; Yates 2015.

10 Bashir et al. 2013.

11 Henry 2013, 162; Inés Taracena 2021.

12 Lehrer 1965.

13 Roosevelt 1933.

14 Aurelius, Epictetus, and Seneca 2014, 42.

15 Milton 2005, 24.

16 Roosevelt 1933.

17 Roosevelt 1933.

18 Kennedy 1968. Parts of this speech can be heard at https://www.youtube.com/watch?v=mCH3KvcAf9w.

19 Pardo 2019.

20 *BBC News* 2020b.

21 https://www.economist.com/leaders/2020/04/23/after-the-disease-the-debt.

22 Strange 1997.

23 Gabor 2020; Kelton 2020.

24 *Economist* 2020c; International Labour Organization 2021.

25 Beck 1999.

26 Chua 2018.

27 García Márquez 1998.

28 García Márquez 1987.

29 *Boston Globe* 2014.

30 Osorio 1991.

31 Osorio 1991.

32 Osorio 1991.

33 Countercurrents Collective 2020.

34 OECD 2020.

35 Kenworthy and Smeeding 2013.

36 Stevis-Grindneff 2020.

37 https://cepi.net; Finn 2020.

38 Allain 2020.

39 Nelson 2009; Perkins and Kuiper 2005.

40 Soper 1995; Conley 1997; Sandilands 1999; Thompson 2006.

41 Collins and Flynn 2008; Martínez-Alier 2012.

42 Curry 2006, 48.

43 Curry 2006, 48.

44 Roser-Renouf et al. 2014; Giddens 1990.

45 Meyerson and Harburg 1993.

46 Gordon Nembhard 2014; Smith 2007; Vickery and Hunter 2014.

47 Schreiber et al. 2013; Zavall, Markowitz, and Weber 2015.

48 Plato 1972.

49 Plato 1972.

50 Bacon 2016.

51 Burke 2003, 603.

52 Burke 2003, 603.

53 Burke 2003, 603.

54 Bentham 1970.

Chapter 4: The Charter

1 MacKenzie 2014, 1, 3.

2 Marx and Engels 1970.

3 Dyson et al. 1994.

4 Lyon 1999, 9.

5 Fassbender 2009.

6 Zetterquist 2011.

7 Gómez and Gasper 2013.

8 Gómez and Gasper 2013.

9 Council of Europe 2020.

10 https://www.ushmm.org/information/exhibitions/online-exhibitions/special-focus/doctors-trial/nuremberg-code#Permissible; https://www.wma.net/policies-post/wma-declaration-of-helsinki-ethical-principles-for-medical-research-involving-human-subjects/; https://www.who.int/medicines/areas/policy/doha_declaration/en/.

11 Flacks and Lichtenstein 2015.

12 AEC 1954.

13 *Scientific American* 2020.

14 *Nature* 2020a.

15 *EClinicalMedicine* 2020.

16 Pūras et al. 2020.

17 WHO 2020b, 2020c.

18 *New England Journal of Medicine* 2020.

19 Chabner et al. 2021.

20 *Lancet Global Health* 2020; UNAIDS 2020.

21 Sliwa and Yacoub 2020.

22 Wabnitz et al. 2020.

23 Hippocrates 2015, 172–173.

24 WHO 2020b.

25 WHO 2020c.

26 Bárcena and Reed 2020.

27 Jolivet et al. 2020.

28 European Commission 2020.

29 UNICEF 2020.

30 COVID-19 Global Solidarity Coalition 2020.

31 OpenDemocracy 2020.

32 AstraZeneca 2020.

33 Baden et al. 2020.

34 U.S. National Academies of Sciences, Engineering, and Medicine 2020.

35 *Economist* 2020c.

36 Marx 1951, 14.

37 Chatzidakis et al. 2020, 10.

38 Chatzidakis et al. 2020, 101.

39 YouTube 2013.

Acknowledgments

1 Pepys 2000, 17.

2 Defoe 2012, 1586.

3 Camus 1948, 254.

References

Adhanom Ghebreyesus, Tedros. 2020. "Going It Alone Will Perpetuate the Economic and Health Crisis—for All." *Economist*, September 8, 2020. https://www.economist.com/by-invitation/2020/09/08/tedros-adhanom-on-why-vaccine-nationalism-harms-efforts-to-halt-the-pandemic.

———. 2021. "WHO Director-General's Opening Remarks at 148th Session of the Executive Board." WHO, January 18, 2021. https://www.who.int/director-general/speeches/detail/who-director-general-s-opening-remarks-at-148th-session-of-the-executive-board.

Adorno, Theodor W. 1975. "Culture Industry Reconsidered." Translated by Anson G. Rabinbach. *New German Critique* 7:12–19.

Advani, Arun, George Bangham, and Jack Leslie. 2021. *The UK's Wealth Distribution and Characteristics of High-Wealth Households*. Resolution Foundation. https://www.resolutionfoundation.org/publications/the-uks-wealth-distribution-and-characteristics-of-high-wealth-households/.

AEC (United States Atomic Energy Commission). 1954. "In the Matter of J. Robert Oppenheimer. Transcript of Hearing Before Personnel Security Board." https://www.osti.gov/opennet/hearing.

AFP, and Christian Borbon. 2020. "Coronavirus Panic Buying: The Psychology behind Toilet Paper Hoarding." *Gulf News*, March 17, 2020. https://gulfnews.com/photos/news/coronavirus

-panic-buying-the-psychology-behind-toilet-paper-hoarding-1 .1584423699719?slide=1.

Agamben, Giorgio. 2009. *What Is an Apparatus? And Other Essays*. Translated by David Kishik and Stefan Pedatella. Stanford: Stanford University Press.

Agren, David. 2020. "Mexican President López Obrador Draws Doctors' Ire." *Lancet* 395, no. 10237: 1601.

Ahmad, Tauseef, and Jin Hui. 2020. "One Health Approach and Coronavirus Disease 2019." *Human Vaccines & Immunotherapeutics* 16, no. 4: 931–932.

Akiyama, Matthew J., Anne C. Spaulding, and Josiah D. Rich. 2020. "Flattening the Curve for Incarcerated Populations—Covid-19 in Jails and Prisons." *New England Journal of Medicine* 382:2075–2077.

Allain, Rhett. 2020. "The Promising Math behind 'Flattening the Curve.'" *Wired*, March 24, 2020. https://www.wired.com/story/the -promising-math-behind-flattening-the-curve/.

Allcott, Hunt, and Matthew Gentzkow. 2017. "Social Media and Fake News in the 2016 Election." *Journal of Economic Perspectives* 31, no. 2: 211–236.

Allier-Montaño, Eugenia, and Emilio Crenzel, eds. 2015. *The Struggle for Memory in Latin America: Recent History and Political Violence*. New York: Palgrave Macmillan.

Alsema, Adriaan. 2020. "Colombia's Health Minister Blaming Hospitals for Coronavirus Chaos." *Colombia Reports*, June 7, 2020. https://colombiareports.com/health-minister-blaming-hospitals -for-colombias-coronavirus-chaos/.

Althusser, Louis. 1969. *For Marx*. Translated by Ben Brewster. Harmondsworth: Penguin.

Amariles, Pedro, Johan Granados, Mauricio Ceballos, and Carlos Julio Montoya. 2021. "COVID-19 in Colombia Endpoints. Are We Different, Like Europe?" *Research in Social and Administrative Pharmacy* 17, no. 1: 2036–2039.

Americans for Tax Fairness and Institute for Policy Studies. 2020. *National Billionaires Report*. https://docs.google.com/spreadsheets/

d/1qLbVmE3QyBho6GFFYkUv7eEWvz8DInZam4dx5vyLtT8/edit#gid=1259834744.

Amnesty International. 2020. "Policing the Pandemic: Human Rights Violations in the Enforcement of COVID-19 Measures in Europe." June 24, 2020. https://www.amnesty.org/en/documents/eur01/2511/2020/en/.

Andrasfay, Theresa, and Noreen Goldman. 2021. "Reductions in 2020 Life Expectancy Due to COVID-19 and the Disproportionate Impact on the Black and Latino Populations." *PLoS* 118, no. 5: e2014746118.

Angel, Arturo. 2021. "En México asesinaron a más de 35 mil personas en 2020, solo un 0.4% menos que un año antes." *Animal Político*, January 21, 2021. https://www.animalpolitico.com/2021/01/mexico-homicidios-35-mil-2020/.

Animal Político. 2017. "Distribución de la riqueza, obstáculo que impide la igualdad social en México: CEPAL." May 30, 2017. https://www.animalpolitico.com/2017/05/distribucion-riqueza-desigualdad-cepal/.

———. 2020. "Obesidad y muertes por COVID: Salud llama a un cambio radical de alimentación." July 23, 2020. https://www.animalpolitico.com/2020/07/obesidad-y-muertes-por-covid-salud-llama-a-un-cambio-radical-de-alimentacion/.

Anshelm, Jonas, and Martin Hultman. 2014. "A Green Fatwā? Climate Change as a Threat to the Masculinity of Industrial Modernity." *NORMA: International Journal of Masculinity Studies* 9, no. 2: 84–96.

Anti-Corruption Resource Centre, Transparency International, and Chr. Michelsen Institute. (2013). *Colombia: Overview of Corruption and Anti-Corruption*. https://knowledgehub.transparency.org/assets/uploads/helpdesk/373_Colombia_Overview_of_corruption_and_anti-corruption.pdf.

APM Research Lab. 2021. "The Color of Coronavirus: COVID-19 Deaths by Race and Ethnicity in the U.S." January 13, 2021. https://www.apmresearchlab.org/covid/deaths-by-race.

Arminen, Illka. 2010. "Who's Afraid of Financial Markets?" *International Sociology* 25, no. 2: 170–183.

Arnold, Catharine. 2018. *Pandemic 1918: Eyewitness Accounts from the Greatest Medical Holocaust in Modern History*. New York: St. Martin's Press.

Arredondo, Armando, and Patricia Nájera. 2008. "Equity and Accessibility in Health? Out-of-Pocket Expenditures on Health Care in Middle Income Countries: Evidence from Mexico." *Cadernos de Saude Publica* 24, no. 12: 2819–2826.

Associated Press. 2020. "One in Every Five Prisoners in US Has Tested Positive for Covid-19." *Guardian*, December 18, 2020. https://www.theguardian.com/us-news/2020/dec/18/us-prisoners-coronavirus-stats-data.

AstraZeneca. 2020. "Biopharma Leaders Unite to Stand with Science." September 8, 2020. https://www.astrazeneca.com/media-centre/press-releases/2020/biopharma-leaders-unite-to-stand-with-science.html.

Aurelius, Marcus, Epictetus, and Seneca. 2014. *Stoic Six Pack: Meditations of Marcus Aurelius, Golden Sayings, Fragments and Discourses of Epictetus, Letters from a Stoic and the Enchiridion*. n.p.: Enhanced Media.

Bacon, Francis. 2016. *New Atlantis and the Great Instauration*. 2nd ed. Edited by Jerry Weinberger. Malden: Wiley-Blackwell.

Baden, Lindsey R., Caren G. Solomon, Michael F. Greene, Ralp B. D'Agostino, and David Harrington. 2020. "The FDA and the Importance of Trust." *New England Journal of Medicine* 383:e148.

Balmori de la Miyar, José Roberto, Lauren Hoehn-Velasco, and Adan Silverio-Murillo. 2020. "Druglords Don't Stay at Home: COVID-19 Pandemic and Crime Patterns in Mexico City." *Journal of Criminal Justice*. https://www.sciencedirect.com/science/article/pii/S0047235220302397?via%3Dihub.

Bank of England. n.d. *Household Credit—a Visual Summary of Our Data*. https://www.bankofengland.co.uk/statistics/visual-summaries/household-credit.

Bárcena, Alicia, and Gail Reed. 2020. "We Are Calling for Adoption of Universal, Redistributive and Solidarity-Based Policies with a Rights-Oriented Approach to Leave No One Behind." *MEDICC Review* 22, no. 2: 8–11.

Barclay, Donald A. 2018. *Fake News, Propaganda, and Plain Old Lies: How to Find Trustworthy Information in the Digital Age*. Lanham, Md.: Rowman & Littlefield.

Baron, Jonathan. 2006. *Against Bioethics*. Cambridge, Mass.: MIT Press.

Barraza-Lloréns, Mariana, Stefano Bertozzi, Eduardo González-Pier, and Juan Pablo Gutiérrez. 2002. "Addressing Inequity in Health and Health Care in Mexico." *Health Affairs* 21, no. 3: 47–56.

Bashir, Nadia Y., Penelope Lockwood, Alison L. Chasteen, Daniel Nadolny, and Indra Noyes. 2013. "The Ironic Impact of Activists: Negative Stereotypes Reduce Social Change Influence." *European Journal of Social Psychology* 43, no. 7: 614–626.

Baudrillard, Jacques. 1988. *Selected Writings*. Edited by Mark Poster. Stanford: Stanford University Press.

BBC News. 2020a. "Coronavirus: Crime Concerns as Disruption Widens." March 24, 2020. https://www.bbc.com/news/uk-wales-52019550.

———. 2020b. "Thousands Join Anti-government Protests across Colombia." November 19, 2020. https://www.bbc.com/news/world-latin-america-55009964.

BBC News Mundo. 2018. "Por qué en Colombia sé necesitan 11 generaciones para salir de la pobreza y en Chile 6." August 2, 2018. https://www.bbc.com/mundo/noticias-45022393.

Beck, Ulrich. 1999. *World Risk Society*. Cambridge, Mass.: Polity Press.

Becker, Gary S. 1993. *Human Capital: A Theoretical and Empirical Analysis with Special Reference to Education*. 3rd ed. Chicago: University of Chicago Press.

Bentham, Jeremy. 1970. *The Principles of Morals and Legislation*. Darien: Hafner.

Bhala, Neeraj, Gwenetta Curry, Adrian R. Martineau, Charles Agyemang, and Raj Bhopal. 2020. "Sharpening the Global Focus on Ethnicity and Race in the Time of COVID-19." *Lancet* 395, no. 10238: P1673–P1676.

Bhattacharya, Aveek, and Jake Shepherd. 2020. *Measuring and Mitigating Child Hunger in the UK*. London: Social Market Foundation.

Biden, Joseph R. 2021. *National Strategy for the COVID-19 Response and Pandemic Preparedness*. https://int.nyt.com/data/documenttools/national-strategy-for-the-covid-19-response/c7bd8ecb9308d669/full.pdf.

Blanchett, Cate. 2020. "Covid-19 Has Ravaged the Whole Idea of Small Government." *Guardian*, October 28, 2020. https://www.theguardian.com/books/2020/oct/29/cate-blanchett-covid-19-has-ravaged-the-whole-idea-of-small-government.

Blanchflower, David G., and Andrew J. Oswald. 2020. "Trends in Extreme Distress in the United States, 1993–2019." *American Journal of Public Health* 110, no. 10: 1538–1544.

Boseley, Sarah. 2021. "Reasons Why Covid Variant Could Kill More People Are Uncertain." *Guardian*, January 22, 2021. https://www.theguardian.com/world/2021/jan/22/reasons-why-covid-variant-could-kill-more-people-are-uncertain.

Boston Globe. 2014. "Gabriel Garcia Marquez Case Shows Need to Let Critics Visit Us." April 19, 2014. https://www.bostonglobe.com/opinion/editorials/2014/04/18/gabriel-garcia-marquez-case-shows-need-let-critics-visit/FIOHyDTHgASoYXcHIFeNmK/story.html.

Bourdieu, Pierre. 1998. *Acts of Resistance: Against the New Myths of Our Time*. Translated by Richard Nice. Cambridge, Mass.: Polity Press.

Boykoff, Maxwell T., and Tom Yulsman. 2013. "Political Economy, Media, and Climate Change: Sinews of Modern Life." *WIREs Climate Change*. http://sciencepolicy.colorado.edu/admin/publication_files/2013.19.pdf.

Bristow, Nancy K. 2012. *American Pandemic: The Lost Worlds of the 1918 Influenza Pandemic*. New York: Oxford University Press.

Brown, Wendy. 2019. *In the Ruins of Neoliberalism: The Rise of Anti-democratic Politics in the West*. New York: Columbia University Press.

Bull, Hedley. 2012. *The Anarchical Society: A Study of Order in World Politics*. 4th ed. Houndmills: Palgrave Macmillan.

Burke, Edmund. 2003. *Reflections on the Revolution in France*. Edited by Frank M. Turner. New Haven: Yale University Press.

Burtless, Gary. 2014. "Has Rising Inequality Brought Us Back to the 1920s?" *Up Front Brookings*, May 20, 2014. https://www.brookings.edu/blog/up-front/2014/05/20/has-rising-inequality-brought-us-back-to-the-1920s-it-depends-on-how-we-measure-income/.

Busch, Lawrence, Richard Allison, Craig Harris, Alan Rudy, Bradle T. Shaw, Toby Ten Eyck, Dawn Coppin, Jason Konefal, and Christopher Oliver, with James Fairweather. 2004. *External Review of the Collaborative Research Agreement between Novartis Agricultural Discovery Institute, Inc. and the Regents of the University of California*. East Lansing: Institute for Food and Agricultural Standards, Michigan State University.

Butt, Nathalie, Frances Lambrick, Mary Menton, and Anna Renwick. 2019. "The Supply Chain of Violence." *Nature Sustainability* 2:742–747.

Caiani, Manuela, and Simona Guerra, eds. 2017. *Euroscepticism, Democracy and the Media: Communicating Europe, Contesting Europe*. London: Palgrave Macmillan.

Camhaji, Elías. 2020. "'Vamos a saquearlo todo': Así operan los grupos que incitan a la rapiña por el coronavirus en México." *El País*, March 29, 2020. https://elpais.com/sociedad/2020-03-29/vamos-a-saquearlo-todo-asi-operan-los-grupos-que-incitan-a-la-rapina-por-el-coronavirus-en-mexico.html.

Campbell, Denis. 2020. "UK Scientists Trial Drug to Prevent Infection That Leads to Covid." *Guardian*, December 25, 2020. https://www.theguardian.com/world/2020/dec/25/uk-scientists-trial-drug-to-prevent-coronavirus-infection-leading-to-disease.

Camus, Albert. 1948. *The Plague*. Translated by Stuart Gilbert. New York: Random House.

Canovan, Margaret. 1981. *Populism*. New York: Harcourt Brace Jovanovich.

Caplan, Arthur L., and Robert Arp, eds. 2013. *Contemporary Debates in Bioethics*. Malden: Wiley-Blackwell.

Cárdenas, Enrique, José Antonio Ocampo, and Rosemary Thorp, eds. 2000. *An Economic History of Twentieth-Century Latin America*. Vol. 3, *Industrialization and the State in Latin America: The Postwar Years*. Houndmills: Palgrave.

Carpenter, Zoë. 2020. "What We Know about the Covid-19 Race Gap." *Nation*, May 4, 2020. https://www.thenation.com/article/society/covid-19-racial-disparities/.

Carr, Edward Hallett. 1964. *The Twenty Years' Crisis, 1919–1939: An Introduction to the Study of International Relations*. New York: Harper Perennial.

Case, Anne, and Angus Deaton. 2020. *Deaths of Despair and the Future of Capitalism*. Princeton: Princeton University Press.

Castro, Carolina, María de Pilar López Uribe, Fernando Posada, Bhavani Castro, and Roudabeh Kishi. 2020. "Understanding the Killing of Social Leaders in Colombia During Covid 19." LSE Latin America and Caribbean, October 6, 2020. https://blogs.lse.ac.uk/latamcaribbean/2020/10/06/understanding-the-killing-of-social-leaders-in-colombia-during-covid-19/.

CDC. 2021. "Allergic Reactions Including Anaphylaxis after Receipt of the First Dose of Pfizer-BioNTech COVID-19 Vaccine—United States, December 14–23, 2020." *Mobility and Mortality Weekly Report* 70:1–6.

Cele, S., I. Gazy, L. Jackson, S.-H. Hwa, H. Tegally, G. Lustig, J. Giandhari, S. Pillay, E. Wilkinson, Y. Naidoo, F. Karim, Y. Ganga, K. Khan, A. B. Balazs, B. I. Gosnell, W. Hanekom, M. Y. S. Moosa, NGS-SA, COMMIT-KZN Team, R. Lessells, T. de Oliveira, and A. Sigal. 2021. "Escape of SARS-CoV-2 501Y.V2 Variants from Neutralization by Convalescent Plasma."

medRxiv. https://www.ahri.org/wp-content/uploads/2021/01/MEDRXIV-2021-250224v1-Sigal.pdf.

Chabner, Bruce A., Susan E. Bates, Antonio Tito Fojo, Ann Murphy, A. Oliver Sartor, and Martin J. Murphy. 2021. "A Medical Pearl Harbor: Pandemic Uncovers Societal Fissures and Leadership Breaches." *Oncologist* 25, no. 1. https://theoncologist.onlinelibrary.wiley.com/doi/pdf/10.1002/onco.13677.

Chakrabortty, Aditya. 2019. "Britain's Infrastructure Is Breaking Down. And Here's Why No One's Fixing It." *Guardian*, August 14, 2019. https://www.theguardian.com/commentisfree/2019/aug/14/britain-social-infrastructure-money-national-grid.

———. 2020a. "Care Workers with Coronavirus Face an Awful Choice: Live in Poverty or Risk Killing Your Patient." *Guardian*, July 9, 2020. https://www.theguardian.com/commentisfree/2020/jul/09/care-workers-coronavirus-poverty-sickness-statutory-sick-pay.

———. 2020b. "England's Test and Trace Is a Fiasco Because the Public Sector Has Been Utterly Sidelined." *Guardian*, September 17, 2020. https://www.theguardian.com/commentisfree/2020/sep/17/england-test-and-trace-public-sector-boris-johnson-covid.

———. 2020c. "The Left Is Not Dead. Britain Is Still Crying Out for a Radical Alternative." *Guardian*, September 3, 2020. https://www.theguardian.com/commentisfree/2020/sep/03/left-britain-radical-alternative-injustice-progressive-reform.

———. 2020d. "Right Now, the Only Thing Staving off a Collapse in the Social Order Is the State." *Guardian*, May 13, 2020. https://www.theguardian.com/commentisfree/2020/may/13/state-collapse-social-order-coronavirus-britain.

———. 2020e. "There's a Hidden Epidemic of Racism in UK Schools—but It's Finally Coming to Light." *Guardian*, July 22, 2020. https://www.theguardian.com/commentisfree/2020/jul/22/racism-uk-schools-teenager.

Chapin, Christy Ford. 2015. *Ensuring America's Health: The Public Creation of the Corporate Health Care System*. New York: Cambridge University Press.

Chappell, Bill. 2020. "'The Vaccine Is on Its Way, Folks,' Fauci Says as Brooklyn Names Him a COVID-19 Hero." *NPR*, November 10, 2020. https://www.npr.org/sections/coronavirus-live-updates/2020/11/10/933439300/the-vaccines-on-its-way-folks-fauci-says-as-brooklyn-names-him-a-covid-hero.

Chatzidakis, Andreas, Jamie Hakim, Jo Littler, Catherine Rottenberg, and Lynne Segal. 2020. *The Care Manifesto: The Politics of Interdependence*. London: Verso.

Cherniavsky, Eva. 2017. *Neocitizenship: Political Culture after Democracy*. New York: New York University Press.

Christensen, Jens H. E., Eric Fischer, and Patrick J. Shultz. 2020. "Emerging Bond Markets and COVID-19: Evidence from Mexico." FRBSF Economic Letter, August 17, 2020. https://www.frbsf.org/economic-research/publications/economic-letter/2020/august/emerging-bond-markets-and-covid-19-evidence-from-mexico/.

Chua, Amy. 2018. *Day of Empire: How Hyperpowers Rise to Global Dominance—and Why They Fall*. New York: Anchor.

CIA. 2020. *The World Factbook*. Accessed October 10, 2020. https://www.cia.gov/the-world-factbook/.

Cifuentes, Myriam Patricia, Laura A. Rodriguez-Villamizar, Maylen Liseth Rojas-Botero, Carlos Alvarez-Moreno, and Julián A. Fernández-Niño. 2020. "Socioeconomic Inequalities Associated with Mortality for COVID-19 in Colombia: A Cohort Nation-Wide Study." *medRxiv*. https://www.medrxiv.org/content/10.1101/2020.12.14.20248203v1.

Claude, Inis. 1971. *Swords into Ploughshares*. New York: Random House.

Coalition for Epidemic Preparedness Innovations, Gavi, and WHO. 2021. *COVAX Global Supply Forecast*. January 20, 2021. https://www.gavi.org/sites/default/files/covid/covax/COVAX%20Supply%20Forecast.pdf.

Coker, Richard. 2020. "'Harvesting' Is a Terrible Word—but It's What Has Happened in Britain's Care Homes." *Guardian*, May 8, 2020. https://www.theguardian.com/commentisfree/2020/may/08/care

-home-residents-harvested-left-to-die-uk-government-herd-immunity.
Cole, Luke W., and Sheila R. Foster. 2001. *From the Ground Up: Environmental Racism and the Rise of the Environmental Justice Movement*. New York: New York University Press.
Collins, Andrea, and David Flynn. 2008. "Measuring the Environmental Sustainability of a Major Sporting Event: A Case Study of the FA Cup Final." *Tourism Economics* 14, no. 4: 751–768.
Collyns, Dan, Sam Cowie, Joe Parkin Daniels, and Tom Phillips. 2020. "'Coronavirus Could Wipe Us Out': Indigenous South Americans Blockade Villages." *Guardian*, March 30, 2020. https://www.theguardian.com/world/2020/mar/30/south-america-indigenous-groups-coronavirus-brazil-colombia.
Conley, Verena Andermatt. 1997. *Ecopolitics: The Environment in Poststructuralist Thought*. London: Routledge.
Correia, Sergio, Stephan Luck, and Emil Verner. 2020. "Pandemics Depress the Economy, Public Health Interventions Do Not: Evidence from the 1918 Flu." http://dx.doi.org/10.2139/ssrn.3561560.
Cosgrove, Ben. 1969. "Faces of the American Dead in Vietnam: One Week's Toll, June 1969." *Life*, June 27, 1969. https://www.life.com/history/faces-of-the-american-dead-in-vietnam-one-weeks-toll-june-1969/.
Council of Europe. 2020. "Social Rights in Times of Pandemic." Accessed October 10, 2020. https://www.coe.int/en/web/european-social-charter/social-rights-in-times-of-pandemic.
Countercurrents Collective. 2020. "Coronavirus Pandemic: China and Cuba Send Medical Teams, Equipment and Medicine to Countries." *Pressenza*, March 19, 2020. https://www.pressenza.com/2020/03/coronavirus-pandemic-china-and-cuba-send-medical-teams-equipment-and-medicine-to-countries/.
COVID-19 Global Solidarity Coalition. 2020. "COVID-19 Global Solidarity Manifesto." April 19, 2020. https://www.covidglobalsolidarity.org.

Cowley, Stacy. 2021. "Vaccine Critics Received More Than $1 Million in Pandemic Relief Loans." *New York Times*, January 18, 2021. https://www.nytimes.com/2021/01/18/business/anti-vaccine-ppp-loans.html.

Cox, Robert W., and Harold Karan Jacobson, eds. 1974. *The Anatomy of Influence: Decision Making in International Organization*. New Haven: Yale University Press.

Curini, Luigi. 2018. *Corruption, Ideology, and Populism: The Rise of Valence Political Campaigning*. Cham: Palgrave Macmillan.

Curry, Patrick. 2006. *Ecological Ethics: An Introduction*. Cambridge, Mass.: Polity Press.

Cyranoski, David. 2021. "Alarming COVID Variants Show Vital Role of Genomic Surveillance." *Nature* 589:337–338.

Dal-Ré, Rafael, Walter Orenstein, and Arthur L. Caplan. 2021. "Trial Participants' Rights after Authorisation of COVID-19." *Lancet Respiratory Medicine*, January 18, 2021. https://www.thelancet.com/journals/lanres/article/PIIS2213-2600(21)00044-8/fulltext.

Daskal, Jennifer. 2020. "Digital Surveillance Can Help Bring the Coronavirus Pandemic under Control—but Also Threatens Privacy." *Conversation*, April 13, 2020. https://theconversation.com/digital-surveillance-can-help-bring-the-coronavirus-pandemic-under-control-but-also-threatens-privacy-135151.

Davidson, Donald. 2004. *Problems of Rationality*. Oxford: Clarendon Press.

Davis, Mike. 2020. *The Monster Enters: COVID-19, Avian Flu, and the Plagues of Capitalism*. New York: OR Books.

Defoe, Daniel. 2012. *Complete Works of Daniel Defoe*. Hastings: Delphi.

De La Torre, Carlos, ed. 2015. *The Promise and Perils of Populism: Global Perspectives*. Lexington: University of Kentucky Press.

Desli, Evangelia, and Alexandra Gkoulgkoutsika. 2020. "Military Spending and Economic Growth: A Panel Data Investigation." *Economic Change and Restructuring*. https://doi.org/10.1007/s10644-020-09267-8.

Deutsche Welle. 2021. "Restaurantes de CDMX: Abrir o morir." January 16, 2021. https://www.dw.com/es/restaurantes-de-cdmx-abrir-o-morir/av-56245770.

Diss, Kathryn. 2020. "Preppers Were Considered Foolish Doomsayers before Coronavirus. Now They Feel Vindicated." *ABC News*, March 28, 2020. https://www.abc.net.au/news/2020-03-28/coronavirus-fears-see-americans-stockpile-guns/12088298.

Dlamini, Judy. 2020. "Gender-Based Violence, Twin Pandemic to COVID-19." *Critical Sociology*. https://doi.org/10.1177/0896920520975465.

Dorling, Daniel. 2013. *Unequal Health: The Scandal of Our Times*. Bristol: Policy Press.

———. 2014. *Inequality and the 1%*. London: Verso.

Doucleff, Michaeleen. 2020. "Why Poorer Countries Aren't Likely to Get the Pfizer Vaccine Any Time Soon." *NPR*, November 11, 2020. https://www.npr.org/sections/goatsandsoda/2020/11/11/933942711/why-poorer-countries-arent-likely-to-get-the-pfizer-vaccine-any-time-soon?utm_source=twitter.com&utm_medium=social&utm_term=nprnews&utm_campaign=npr.

Dow, Eddy. 1988. "The Rich Are Different." *New York Times*, November 13, 1988, 70.

Dunlap, Riley E., and Peter J. Jacques. 2013. "Climate Change Denial Books and Conservative Think Tanks: Exploring the Connection." *American Behavioral Scientist* 57, no. 6: 699–731.

Dyson, Esther, George Gilder, George Keyworth, and Alvin Toffler. 1994. "Cyberspace and the American Dream: A Magna Carta for the Knowledge Age." Version 1.2. Progress and Freedom Foundation. Accessed October 10, 2020. http://www.pff.org/issues-pubs/futureinsights/fi1.2magnacarta.html.

Ebrahim, Shahul H., and Ziad A. Memish. 2020. "COVID-19: Preparing for Superspreader Potential among Umrah Pilgrims to Saudi Arabia." *Lancet* 395, no. 10227: e48.

ECLAC (Economic Commission for Latin America and the Caribbean). 2019. "Social Panorama of Latin America 2018."

February 2019. https://www.cepal.org/en/publications/44396-social-panorama-latin-america-2018.

EClinicalMedicine. 2020. "Dear Mr. President, You Can't Lie Your Way Out of This Pandemic!" 27, no. 100619. https://www.thelancet.com/journals/eclinm/article/PIIS2589-5370(20)30363-1/fulltext.

Economist. 2006. "The Rich, the Poor and the Growing Gap between Them." June 15, 2006. https://www.economist.com/special-report/2006/06/15/the-rich-the-poor-and-the-growing-gap-between-them.

———. 2020a. "The Pandemic Further Weakens Latin America's Underperforming Schools." September 12, 2020. https://www.economist.com/the-americas/2020/09/12/the-pandemic-further-weakens-latin-americas-underperforming-schools.

———. 2020b. "Pfizer's and BioNTech's Vaccine Is the Start of the End of the Pandemic." November 9, 2020. https://www.economist.com/science-and-technology/2020/11/09/pfizers-and-biontechs-vaccine-is-the-start-of-the-end-of-the-pandemic.

———. 2020c. "The Plague Year." December 19, 2020.

———. 2021a. "China's Economy Zooms Back to Its Pre-Covid Rate." January 18, 2021. https://www.economist.com/finance-and-economics/2021/01/18/chinas-economy-zooms-back-to-its-pre-covid-growth-rate.

———. 2021b. "Commodity Prices Are Surging." January 16, 2021. https://www.economist.com/finance-and-economics/2021/01/12/commodity-prices-are-surging.

———. 2021c. "Have Banks Got Too Much Cash?" January 20, 2021. https://www.economist.com/finance-and-economics/2021/01/20/have-banks-now-got-too-much-cash.

Economist Intelligence Unit, Nuclear Threat Initiative, and Johns Hopkins Bloomberg School of Public Health Center for Health Security. 2019. "Global Health Security Index: Building Collective Action and Accountability." October 2019. https://www.ghsindex.org/wp-content/uploads/2020/04/2019-Global-Health-Security-Index.pdf.

Eisenhower, Dwight D. 1961. "Transcript of President Dwight D. Eisenhower's Farewell Address (1961)." Our Documents. Accessed October 10, 2020. https://www.ourdocuments.gov/doc.php?flash=false&doc=90&page=transcript.

EIU (Economist Intelligence Unit). 2019. "Colombia: Fact Sheet." May 1, 2019. http://country.eiu.com/article.aspx?articleid=1048240888&Country=Colombia&topic=Summary&subtopic=Fact+sheet.

El Tiempo. 2020. "Covid-19 deja 176 muertes más y 6.731 casos nuevos en Colombia." September 23, 2020. https://www.eltiempo.com/salud/coronavirus-en-colombia-muertes-y-contagios-23-de-septiembre-del-2020-539474.

Emanuel, Ezekiel J., Govind Persad, Ross Upshur, Beatriz Thome, Michael Parker, Aaron Glickman, Cathy Zhang, Connor Boyle, Maxwell Smith, and James P. Phillips. 2020. "Fair Allocation of Scarce Medical Resources in the Time of Covid-19." *New England Journal of Medicine* 382:2049–2055.

Emanuel, Ezekiel J., Cathy Zhang, Aaron Glickman, Emily Gudbranson, Sarah S. P. DiMagno, and John W. Urwin. 2020. "Drug Reimbursement Regulation in 6 Peer Countries." *JAMA Internal Medicine* 180, no. 11: 1510–1517.

Emmison, Mike. 1983. "'The Economy': Its Emergence in Media Discourse." In *Language, Image, Media*, edited by Howard Davis and Paul Walton, 139–155. Oxford: Basil Blackwell.

Emmison, Mike, and Alec McHoul. 1987. "Drawing on the Economy: Cartoon Discourse and the Production of a Category." *Cultural Studies* 1, no. 1: 93–111.

Engels, Friedrich. 1893. "Engels to Franz Mehring." Letter, July 14, 1893. Translated by Donna Torr. Marxists Internet Archive. https://www.marxists.org/archive/marx/works/1893/letters/93_07_14.htm.

———. 1946. *The Dialectics of Nature*. Edited and translated by Clemens Dutt. London: Lawrence & Wishart.

European Commission. 2020. "Manifesto for EU COVID-19 Research: Maximising the Accessibility of Research Results in the Fight against COVID-19." https://ec.europa.eu/info/

research-and-innovation/research-area/health-research-and-innovation/coronavirus-research-and-innovation/covid-research-manifesto_en.

Faculty of Intensive Care Medicine. 2017. *A Report on the First Wave Survey*. https://www.ficm.ac.uk/sites/default/files/critical_futures_2017_0.pdf.

Fassbender, Bardo. 2009. *The United Nations Charter as the Constitution of the International Community*. Leiden: Koninklijke Brill.

FBI. 2019. "Crime in the United States, 2019: Expanded Homicide Data." https://ucr.fbi.gov/crime-in-the-u.s/2019/crime-in-the-u.s.-2019/topic-pages/expanded-homicide.pdf.

Ferri, Pablo. 2020a. "México vive su mes más violento pese a la pandemia." *El País*, April 2, 2020. https://elpais.com/internacional/2020-04-02/mexico-vive-su-mes-mas-violento-pese-a-la-pandemia.html.

———. 2020b. "El narco mexicano aprovecha el virus para exhibir su poder ante las cámaras." *El País*, April 17, 2020. https://elpais.com/internacional/2020-04-17/el-narco-mexicano-aprovecha-el-virus-para-exhibir-su-poder-ante-las-camaras.html.

Fine, Ben, and Juan Pablo Durán Ortiz. 2016. "Social Capital: From the Gringo's Tale to the Colombian Reality." SOAS Department of Economics, Working Paper No. 195, May 2016. https://www.soas.ac.uk/economics/research/workingpapers/file112410.pdf.

Finn, Adam. 2020. "Ten Reasons We Got Covid-19 Vaccines So Quickly without 'Cutting Corners.'" *Guardian*, December 26, 2020. https://www.theguardian.com/commentisfree/2020/dec/26/ten-reasons-we-got-covid-19-vaccines-so-quickly-without-cutting-corners.

Fitzgerald, F. Scott. 1926. "The Rich Boy." Project Gutenberg Australia. http://gutenberg.net.au/fsf/THE-RICH-BOY.html.

Flacks, Richard, and Nelson Lichtenstein, eds. 2015. *The Port Huron Statement: Sources and Legacies of the New Left's Founding Manifesto*. Philadelphia: University of Pennsylvania Press.

Flamand, Laura. 2020. "Federalism and COVID: Managing the Health and Economic Crisis in the Mexican Federation." *Cuadernos Manuel Giménez Abad* 19:28–29.

Flaming, Daniel, Anthony W. Orlando, Patrick Burns, and Seth Pickens. 2021. "Locked Out: Unemployment and Homelessness in the Covid Economy." *Economic Roundtable: Knowledge for the Greater Good.* https://economicrt.org/publication/locked-out/.

Fogel, Aaron. 1993. "The Prose of Populations and the Magic of Demography." *Western Humanities Review* 47, no. 4: 312–337.

Folbre, Nancy. 2010. "Ethics for Economists." *New York Times,* November 8, 2010. https://economix.blogs.nytimes.com/2010/11/08/ethics-for-economists/.

Forbes Mexico. 2020. "Pfizer celebra éxito de su vacuna contra Covid-19: Es un gran día para la humanidad." November 9, 2020. https://www.forbes.com.mx/negocios-pfizer-celebra-exito-de-su-vacuna-contra-covid-19-es-un-gran-dia-para-la-humanidad/.

Foucault, Michel. 1978. *The History of Sexuality,* Vol. 1, *An Introduction.* Translated by Robert Hurley. New York: Pantheon.

———. 1980. *Power/Knowledge: Selected Interviews & Other Writings, 1972–1977.* Edited by Colin Gordon. New York: Pantheon.

———. 1982. "The Subject and Power." Translated by Leslie Sawyer. *Critical Inquiry* 8, no. 4: 779–795.

———. 1991a. *The Foucault Effect: Studies in Governmentality.* Edited by Graham Burchell, Colin Gordon, and Peter Miller. Harlow: Harvester Wheatsheaf.

———. 1991b. *Remarks on Marx: Conversations with Duccio Trombadori.* Translated by R. J. Goldstein and J. Cascaito. New York: Semiotext(e).

———. 2003. *"Society Must Be Defended": Lectures at the Collège de France, 1975–76.* Translated by David Macey. Edited by Mauro Bertani and Alessandro Fontana. New York: Picador.

———. 2004. *Sécurité, territoire, population.* Paris: Seuil/Gallimard.

———. 2007. "Spaces of Security: The Example of the Town, Lecture of 11th January 1978." Translated by Graham Burchell. *Political Geography* 26, no. 1: 48–56.

———. 2008. *The Birth of Biopolitics: Lectures at the Collège de France, 1978–79*. Translated by Graham Burchell. Edited by Michel Senellart. Houndmills: Palgrave Macmillan.

Fowler, Zachary, Elle Moeller, Lina Roa, Isaac Deneb Castañeda-Alcántara, Tarsicio Uribe-Leitz, John G. Meara, and Arturo Cervantes-Trejo. 2020. "Projected Impact of COVID-19 Mitigation Strategies on Hospital Services in the Mexico City Metropolitan Area." *PLoS ONE* 15, no. 11: e024195.

France 24. 2020. "Coronavirus Could Drive Final Nail in Mink Fur Trade." October 18, 2020. https://www.fr24news.com/a/2020/10/coronavirus-could-drive-final-nail-in-mink-fur-trade.html.

Franco-Paredes, Carlos Nazgol Ghandnoosh, Hassan Latif, Martin Krsak, Andres F. Henao-Martinez, Megan Robins, Lilian Vargas Barahona, and Eric M. Poeschla. 2020. "Decarceration and Community Re-entry in the COVID-19 Era." *Lancet Infectious Diseases* 21, no. 1: E11–E16.

Frenk, Julio, and Suerie Moon. 2013. "Governance Challenges in Global Health." *New England Journal of Medicine* 368:936–942.

Friedman, Milton, and Rose D. Friedman. 2002. *Capitalism and Freedom: 40th Anniversary Edition*. Chicago: University of Chicago Press.

Fugh-Berman, Adriane. 2005. "The Corporate Coauthor." *Journal of General Internal Medicine* 20:546–548.

Funk, Cary, and Lee Rainie. 2015. "Public and Scientists' Views on Science and Society." *Pew Research Center*, January 29, 2015. http://www.pewinternet.org/2015/01/29/public-and-scientists-views-on-science-and-society/.

Gabor, Daniela. 2020. "Claims the UK Has 'Maxed Out' Its Credit Card Are Bad Economics." *Guardian*, November 26, 2020. https://www.theguardian.com/commentisfree/2020/nov/26/uk-maxed-out-credit-card-bad-economics-pandemic-austerity.

García Canclini, Néstor. 2020. "¿Llegará el coronavirus a aplastar las demás luchas en curso?" *Clarín*, April 10, 2020. https://www.clarin.com/revista-enie/-revolucion-mundial-_0_4pX-ZaJL7.html.

García Márquez, Gabriel. 1987. *La mala hora*. https://www.cobachsonora.edu.mx/bibliotecacobach/files/libros/Gabriel_Garcia_Marquez_La_mala_hora.pdf.

———. 1998. *Por un país al alcance de los niños*. 2nd ed. Bogotá: Villegas Editores.

Gardner, Jodi, Mia Gray, and Katharina Moser, eds. 2020. *Debt and Austerity: Implications of the Financial Crisis*. Cheltenham: Edward Elgar.

Gearin, Mary, and Ben Knight. 2020. "Family Violence Perpetrators Using COVID-19 as 'a Form of Abuse We Have Not Experienced Before.'" *ABC News*, March 29, 2020. https://www.abc.net.au/news/2020-03-29/coronavirus-family-violence-surge-in-victoria/12098546.

Germain, Sabrina. 2020. "Will COVID-19 Mark the End of an Egalitarian National Health Service?" *European Journal of Risk Regulation* 11:358–365.

Giddens, Anthony. 1990. *The Consequences of Modernity*. Cambridge, Mass.: Polity Press.

Giménez, Víctor, William Prieto, Diego Prior, and Emili Tortosa-Ausina. 2019. "Evaluation of Efficiency in Colombian Hospitals: An Analysis for the Post-Reform Period." *Socio-Economic Planning Sciences* 65, no. 1: 20–35.

Giraldo Durán, Angélica, and Adrián Gutiérrez Álvarez de Castillo. 2018. "Violencia y paz en Colombia: Una mirada desde la reproducción del capital en América Latina." *Interdisciplina* 6, no. 15: 61–81.

Global Witness. 2019. "Enemies of the State?" July 30, 2019. https://www.globalwitness.org/en/campaigns/environmental-activists/enemies-state/.

Godoy, Emilio. 2020. "Mayan Train Threatens to Alter the Environment and Communities in Mexico." *Inter Press Service*, August 25, 2020.

http://www.ipsnews.net/2020/08/mayan-train-threatens-alter-environment-communities-mexico/.
Golding, William. 1954. *Lord of the Flies*. London: Faber & Faber.
Gómez, Oscar A., and Des Gasper. 2013. "Human Security: A Thematic Guidance Note for Regional and National Human Development Report Teams." United Nations Development Programme. http://hdl.handle.net/1765/50571.
Gorbachev, Mikhail. 2009. "Bring Back the State." *New Perspectives Quarterly* 26, no. 2: 53–55.
Gordon Nembhard, Jessica. 2014. *Collective Courage: A History of African American Cooperative Economic Thought and Practice*. University Park: Pennsylvania State University Press.
Government of Canada / Gouvernement du Canada. n.d. "Procuring Vaccines for COVID-19." https://www.canada.ca/en/public-services-procurement/services/procuring-vaccines-covid19.html.
Grady, Denise. 2020. "Early Data Show Moderna's Coronavirus Vaccine Is 94.5% Effective." *New York Times*, November 16, 2020. https://www.nytimes.com/2020/11/16/health/Covid-moderna-vaccine.html?action=click&module=Top%20Stories&pgtype=Homepage.
Graeber, David. 2002. "The New Anarchists." *New Left Review* 13:61–73.
Gramsci, Antonio. 1971. *Selections from the Prison Notebooks*. Translated by Quentin Hoare and Geoffrey Nowell-Smith. New York: International Publishers.
———. 2000. *The Gramsci Reader: Selected Writings 1916–1935*. Edited by David Forgacs. New York: New York University Press.
Grant, Will. 2020. "Mexico Crime: Could This Become the Bloodiest Year on Record?" *BBC*, July 11, 2020. https://www.bbc.com/news/world-latin-america-53332756.
Griffin, Jo, and Daniela Rivera Antara. 2020. "'Separation by Sex': Gendered Lockdown Fuelling Hate Crime on Streets of Bogotá." *Guardian*, May 8, 2020. https://www.theguardian.com/

global-development/2020/may/08/separation-by-sex-gendered-lockdown-fuelling-hate-on-streets-of-bogota.

Guardian. 2019. "'Incalculable Loss': *New York Times* Covers Front Page with 1,000 Covid-19 Death Notices." May 24, 2019. https://www.theguardian.com/world/2020/may/24/new-york-times-front-page-1000-covid-19-death-notices.

Guillot, Louise. 2021. "The Environmental Impact of Mass Coronavirus Vaccinations." *Politico*, January 15, 2021. https://www.politico.eu/article/mass-coronavirus-vaccinations-environmental-impact-climate-change/.

Guzmán Urrea, María del Pilar. 2016. "Case 1: Priority Setting and Crisis of Public Hospitals in Colombia." In *Public Health Ethics: Cases Spanning the Globe*, edited by Drue H. Barrett, Leonard W. Ortmann, Angus Dawson, Carla Saenz, Andreas Reis, and Gail Bolan, 71–74. Cham: Springer.

Hall, Stuart, Chas Critcher, Tony Jefferson, John Clarke, and Brian Roberts. 2013. *Policing the Crisis: Mugging, the State and Law and Order*. 2nd ed. Houndmills: Palgrave Macmillan.

Hall, Stuart, and Doreen Massey. 2010. "Interpreting the Crisis." In *After the Crash: Reinventing the Left in Britain*, edited by Richar S. Grayson and Jonathan Rutherford, 37–46. London: Soundings / Social Liberal Forum / Compass.

Hall, William J., Mimi V. Chapman, Kent M. Lee, Yesenia M. Merino, Tainayah W. Thomas, B. Keith Payne, Eugenia Eng, Steven H. Day, and Tamera Coyne-Beasley. 2015. "Implicit Racial/Ethnic Bias among Health Care Professionals and Its Influence on Health Care Outcomes: A Systematic Review." *American Journal of Public Health* 105, no. 12: e60–e76.

Handwerker, Elizabeth Weber, Peter B. Meyer, Joseph Piacentini, Michael Schults, and Leo Sveikauskas. 2020. "Employment Recovery in the Wake of the COVID-19 Pandemic." *Monthly Labor Review*, December 2020. https://www.bls.gov/opub/mlr/2020/article/employment-recovery.htm.

Hardin, Garrett. 1968. "The Tragedy of the Commons." *Science* 162, no. 3859: 1243–1248.

Harman, Sophie, Asha Herten-Crabb, Rosemary Morgan, Julia Smith, and Clare Wenham. 2020. "COVID-19 Vaccines and Women's Security." *Lancet*. https://doi.org/10.1016/S0140-6736(20)32727-6.

Harrington, Michael. 1962. *The Other America*. New York: Macmillan.

Hart, P. Sol, and Lauren Feldman. 2014. "Threat without Efficacy? Climate Change on U.S. Network News." *Science Communication* 36, no. 3: 325–351.

Häsler, Barbara, Laura Cornelsen, Houda Bennahi, and Jonathan Rushton. 2014. "A Review of the Metrics for One Health Benefits." *Revue Scientifique et Technique* 33, no. 2: 453–464.

Healy, David, Michael E. Thase, Mary Cannon, Kwame McKenzie, and Andrew Sims. 2003. "Is Academic Psychiatry for Sale?" *British Journal of Psychiatry* 182:388–390.

Hellinger, Daniel C. 2015. *Comparative Politics of Latin America: Democracy at Last?* 2nd ed. New York: Routledge.

Hemingway, Ernest. 2016. *The Complete Works of Ernest Hemingway*. Hastings: Delphi Classics.

Henry, O. 2013. *The Complete Works of O. Henry*. Hastings: Delphi Classics.

Herrera de la Fuente, Carlos. 2016. "El fracaso del neoliberalismo en México." *Aristegui*, March 28, 2016. https://aristeguinoticias.com/2803/mexico/el-fracaso-del-neoliberalismo-en-mexico-articulo-de-carlos-herrera-de-la-fuente/.

Hershberg, Eric, Alexandra Flinn-Palcic, and Christopher Kambhu. 2020. "The COVID-19 Pandemic and Latin American Universities." Center for Latin American & Latino Studies, American University, Washington, D.C., June 2, 2020. https://www.american.edu/centers/latin-american-latino-studies/upload/la-higher-ed-covid-final.pdf.

Hill, Michael. 2012. *The Public Policy Process*. 6th ed. London: Routledge.

Hippocrates. 2015. *The Complete Works of Hippocrates*. Hastings: Delphi Classics.

Hobbes, Thomas. n.d. *Of Man, Being the First Part of Leviathan*. Bartleby.com. http://www.bartleby.com/34/5/13.html.

Hofstadter, Richard. 1966. *The Paranoid Style in American Politics and Other Essays*. New York: Knopf.

Hoggart, Richard. 2009. *The Uses of Literacy: Aspects of Working-Class Life*. Harmondsworth: Penguin.

Honigsbaum, Mark. 2020. *The Pandemic Century: A History of Global Contagion from the Spanish Flu to Covid-19*. New York: Penguin.

Hope, David, and Julian Limberg. 2020. "The Economic Consequences of Major Tax Cuts for the Rich." International Inequalities Institute, London School of Economics and Political Science Working Paper 55, December 2020. http://eprints.lse.ac.uk/107919/.

Hopkin, Jonathan. 2020. *Anti-system Politics: The Crisis of Market Liberalism in Rich Democracies*. New York: Oxford University Press.

Horton, Jake. 2020. "Coronavirus: What Are the Numbers Out of Latin America?" *BBC*, September 22, 2020. https://www.bbc.com/news/world-latin-america-52711458.

Horton, Richard. 2020. "Offline: COVID-19 Is Not a Pandemic." *Lancet* 396:874.

House of Commons Digital, Culture, Media and Sport Committee. 2019. *Disinformation and "Fake News": Final Report Eighth Report of Session 2017–19*. London: House of Commons.

IFARMA, and AIS. 2009. "Precio, disponibilidad y asequilibridad de medicamentos y componentes del precio en Colombia." April 7, 2009. http://www.haiweb.org/medicineprices/surveys/200810CO/sdocs/Colombia_FINAL_report_05_08_09.pdf.

IMF (International Monetary Fund). 2019. *Colombia: Selected Issues*. Country Report No. 19/107, April 29, 2019. https://www.imf.org/en/Publications/CR/Issues/2019/04/29/Colombia-Selected-Issues-46829.

———. 2020a. *Colombia: Staff Report for the 2020 Article IV Consultation*. April 2, 2020. https://www.imf.org/en/Publications/

SPROLLs/Article-iv-staff-reports#sort=%40imfdate %20descending.
———. 2020b. *Mexico: IMF Staff Concluding Statement of the 2020 Article IV Mission*. October 6, 2020. https://www.imf.org/en/News/Articles/2020/10/06/mcs100620-mexico-imf-staff-concluding-statement-of-the-2020-article-iv-mission.
Incat Crowther. 2020. "Incat Crowther Releases Details of Next ShadowCAT Concept." November 23, 2020. http://www.incatcrowther.com/News/incat-crowther-releases-details-of-next-shadowcat-concept.
Independent Panel for Pandemic Preparedness and Response. 2021. *Second Report on Progress: Prepared by the Independent Panel for Pandemic Preparedness and Response for the WHO Executive Board, January 2021*. https://theindependentpanel.org/wp-content/uploads/2021/01/Independent-Panel_Second-Report-on-Progress_Final-15-Jan-2021.pdf.
Inés Taracena, Maria. 2021. "Op-Ed: Save Your Privileged Shock." *Remezcla*, January 8, 2021. https://remezcla.com/features/culture/op-ed-capitol-attack-reactions-global-south-reality/.
Innes, Dave. 2020. "What Has Driven the Rise of In-Work Poverty?" Joseph Rowntree Foundation, February 2, 2020. https://www.jrf.org.uk/report/what-has-driven-rise-work-poverty.
International Commission for the Study of Communication Problems. 1980. *Many Voices One World: Towards a New More Just and More Efficient World Information and Communication Order*. Paris: UNESCO.
International Labour Organization. 2021. *ILO Monitor: COVID-19 and the World of Work*. 7th ed. https://www.ilo.org/wcmsp5/groups/public/---dgreports/---dcomm/documents/briefingnote/wcms_767028.pdf.
Ionescu, Ghiţa, and Ernest Gellner, eds. 1969. *Populism: Its Meanings and National Characteristics*. London: Macmillan.
Jensen, Robert. 2007. "The Digital Provide: Information Technology, Market Performance, and Welfare in the South Indian Fisheries Sector." *Quarterly Journal of Economics* 122, no. 3: 879–924.

Johnson, Jake. 2020. "Trump Refuses to Allow Dr. Fauci to Answer Question on Dangers of Hydroxychoroquine." *CommonDreams*, April 6, 2020. https://www.commondreams.org/news/2020/04/06/really-chilling-moment-trump-refuses-allow-dr-fauci-answer-question-dangers.

Jolivet, R. Rima, Charlotte E. Warren, Pooja Sripad, Elena Ateva, Jewel Gausman, Kate Mitchell, Hagar Palgi Hacker, Emma Sacks, and Ana Langer. 2020. "Upholding Rights under COVID-19: The Respectful Maternity Care Charter." *Health and Human Rights Journal* 1:391–394.

Jones, Alexi. 2020. "New BJS Data." *Prison Policy*, October 30, 2020. https://www.prisonpolicy.org/blog/2020/10/30/prisoners_in_2019/.

Jordan, Douglas, with Terrence Tumpey and Barbara Jester. n.d. "The Deadliest Flu: The Complete Story of the Discovery and Reconstruction of the 1918 Pandemic Virus." Centers for Disease Control and Prevention. https://www.cdc.gov/flu/pandemic-resources/reconstruction-1918-virus.html.

Joseph Rowntree Foundation. 2021. *UK Poverty 2020/21*. https://www.jrf.org.uk/report/uk-poverty-2020-21.

Kant, Immanuel. 2011. *Observations on the Feeling of the Beautiful and Sublime and Other Writings*. Edited by Patrick Frierson and Paul Guyer. Cambridge: Cambridge University Press.

Kaplan, Adiel. 2020. "As Covid Cases Soar, GOP State Lawmakers Keep Fighting to Limit Governors' Power to Respond." *NBC News*, November 14, 2020. https://www.nbcnews.com/politics/politics-news/covid-cases-soar-gop-state-lawmakers-keep-fighting-limit-governors-n1247801.

Keay, Douglas. 1987. "Aids, Education and the Year 2000! Interview with Margaret Thatcher." *Woman's Own*, October 31, 1987, 8–10.

Kelton, Stephanie. 2020. *The Deficit Myth: Modern Monetary Theory and the Birth of the People's Economy*. New York: Public Affairs.

Kennedy, Robert F. 1968. "Remarks at the University of Kansas, March 18, 1968." John F. Kennedy Presidential Library and

Museum. https://www.jfklibrary.org/learn/about-jfk/the-kennedy-family/robert-f-kennedy/robert-f-kennedy-speeches/remarks-at-the-university-of-kansas-march-18-1968.

Kenworthy, Lane, and Timothy Smeeding. 2013. "GINI Growing Inequalities' Impacts: Country Report for the United States." January 2013. http://gini-research.org/system/uploads/443/original/US.pdf?1370077377.

Kevany, Sophie. 2020. "Escaped Infected Danish Mink Could Spread Covid in Wild." *Guardian*, November 27, 2020. https://www.theguardian.com/environment/2020/nov/27/escaped-infected-danish-mink-could-spread-covid-in-wild.

Kevany, Sophie, and Tom Carstensen. 2020. "Covid-19 Mink Variants Discovered in Humans in Seven Countries." *Guardian*, November 18, 2020. https://www.theguardian.com/environment/2020/nov/18/covid-19-mink-variants-discovered-in-humans-in-seven-countries.

Kinder, Molly, and Laura Stateler. 2020. "Amazon and Walmart Have Raked in Billions in Additional Profits during the Pandemic, and Shared Almost None of It with Their Workers." *Brookings*, December 22, 2020. https://www.brookings.edu/blog/the-avenue/2020/12/22/amazon-and-walmart-have-raked-in-billions-in-additional-profits-during-the-pandemic-and-shared-almost-none-of-it-with-their-workers/.

Kinder, Molly, Laura Stateler, and Julia Du. 2020. *Windfall Profits and Deadly Risks: How the Biggest Retail Companies Are Compensating Essential Workers during the COVID-19 Pandemic*. Brookings. https://www.brookings.edu/essay/windfall-profits-and-deadly-risks/.

Kitroeff, Natalie, and Paulina Villegas. 2020. "'It's Not the Virus': Mexico's Broken Hospitals Become Killers, Too." *New York Times*, May 28, 2020. https://www.nytimes.com/2020/05/28/world/americas/virus-mexico-doctors.html.

Knight, Malcolm, Norman Loayza, and Delano Villanueva. 1996. "The Peace Dividend: Military Spending Cuts and Economic

Growth." World Bank Policy Research Working Paper 1577. http://documents.worldbank.org/curated/en/154941468766463442/107507322_20041117142015/additional/multiopage.pdf.

Kollewe, Julia. 2020. "Pfizer and BioNTech Could Make $13bn from Coronavirus Vaccine." *Guardian*, November 11, 2020. https://www.theguardian.com/business/2020/nov/10/pfizer-and-biontech-could-make-13bn-from-coronavirus-vaccine?CMP=Share_iOSApp_Other.

Koren, Marina. 2020. "The Pandemic Is Turning the Natural World Upside Down." *Atlantic*, April 2, 2020. https://www.theatlantic.com/science/archive/2020/04/coronavirus-pandemic-earth-pollution-noise/609316/?utm_source=facebook&utm_medium=social&utm_campaign=share.

Kraus, Michael W., Stéphane Côté, and Dacher Keltner. 2010. "Social Class, Contextualism, and Empathic Accuracy." *Psychological Science* 21, no. 11: 1716–1723.

Kriesi, Hanspeter, and Takis S. Pappas, eds. 2015. *European Populism in the Shadow of the Great Recession*. Colchester: ECPR Press.

Kruse, Kevin M. 2015. *One Nation under God: How Corporate America Invented Christian America*. New York: Basic Books.

Lancet. 2020. "COVID-19 in Latin America: A Humanitarian Crisis." 396, no. 10261: 1463.

Lancet Global Health. 2020. "Decolonising COVID-19." 8, no. 5: E612.

Laqua, Daniel. 2011. "Intellectual Cooperation, the League of Nations, and the Problem of Order." *Journal of Global History* 6, no. 2: 223–247.

Latour, Bruno. 1993. *We Have Never Been Modern*. Translated by Catherine Porter. Cambridge, Mass.: Harvard University Press.

———. 2004. *The Politics of Nature*. Translated by Catherine Porter. Cambridge, Mass.: Harvard University Press.

Lawrence, Felicity, Rob Evans, David Pegg, Caelainn Barr, and Pamela Duncan. 2019. "How the Right's Radical Thinktanks Reshaped the Conservative Party." *Guardian*, November 29, 2019. https://www.theguardian.com/politics/2019/nov/29/rightwing-thinktank-conservative-boris-johnson-brexit-atlas-network.

Leal Filho, Walter, Evangelos Manolas, Anabela Marisa Azul, Ulisse M. Azeiteiro, and Henry McGhie, eds. 2018. *Handbook of Climate Change Communication*. Vols. 1–3. Cham: Springer.

Ledford, Heidi. 2021. "How Can Countries Stretch COVID Vaccine Supplies: Scientists Are Divided over Dosing Strategies." *Nature* 589:182.

Le Fanu, James. 2005. "Confronting an Ill Society." *Journal of the Royal Society of Medicine* 98, no. 7: 332–333.

Lehrer, Tom. 1965. "The Folk Song Army." https://sursumcorda.salemsattic.com/archives/2012/03/09/the-new-folk-song-army.

Levy, Santiago. 2008. *Good Intentions, Bad Outcomes: Social Policy, Informality, and Economic Growth in Mexico*. Washington, D.C.: Brookings Institution Press.

Lewandowsky, Stephan, Naomi Oreskes, James S. Risbey, Ben R. Newell, and Michael Smithson. 2015. "Seepage: Climate Change Denial and Its Effect on the Scientific Community." *Global Environmental Change* 33:1–13.

Lindblom, Charles E. 1980. *The Policy-Making Process*. 2nd ed. Englewood Cliffs: Prentice Hall.

Lockie, Stewart. 2017. "Post-truth Politics and the Social Sciences." *Environmental Sociology* 3, no. 1: 1–5.

Lonergan, Eric, and Mark Blyth. 2020. *Angrynomics*. Newcastle: Agenda.

Luthi, Susannah. 2021. "Amazon's Offering to Help Biden's Vaccine Push. There May Be a Reason Why." *Politico*, January 23, 2021. https://www.politico.com/news/2021/01/23/amazon-covid-vaccine-distribution-461525.

Lyon, Janet. 1999. *Manifestoes: Provocations of the Modern*. Ithaca: Cornell University Press.

Lyotard, Jean-François. 1988. *The Differend: Phrases in Dispute*. Translated by Georges Van Den Abbeele. Minneapolis: University of Minnesota Press.

MacKenzie, Scott, ed. 2014. *Film Manifestos and Global Cinema Cultures: A Critical Anthology*. Berkeley: University of California Press.

Mahase, Elisabeth. 2020. "Covid-19: What Have We Learnt about the New Variant in the UK?" *British Medical Journal* 371:m4944.

Malpas, Jeffrey. 1992. "Retrieving Truth: Modernism, Post-modernism and the Problem of Truth." *Soundings* 75, nos. 2–3: 288–306.

Marcos, Ana. 2016. "El voto evangélico, clave en la victoria del 'no' en el plebiscito de Colombia." *El País*, October 12, 2016. https://elpais.com/internacional/2016/10/12/colombia/1476237985_601462.html.

Marcos Recio, Juan Carlos, Juan Miguel Sánchez Vigil, and María Olivera Zaldua. 2017. "La enorme mentira y la gran verdad de la información en tiempos de la postverdad." *Scire: Representación y organización del conocimiento* 23, no. 2: 13–23.

Marmot, Michael G. 2004. "Evidence Based Policy or Policy Based Evidence?" *British Medical Journal* 328, no. 7445: 906–907.

Martín-Barbero, Jesús. 2001. "Introducción." In *Imaginarios de Nación: Pensar en Medio de la Tormenta*, edited by Jesús Martin-Barbero, 7–10. Bogotá: Ministerio de Cultura.

Martínez-Alier, Joan. 2012. "Environmental Justice and Economic Degrowth: An Alliance between Two Movements." *Capitalism Nature Socialism* 23, no. 1: 51–73.

Marx, Karl. 1951. *The Eighteenth Brumaire of Louis Bonaparte*. Translated by Daniel de Leon. New York: New York Labor News.

———. 1987. *Capital*. Vol. 1, *A Critical Analysis of Capitalist Production*. 3rd ed. Translated by Samuel Moore and Edward Aveling. Edited by Friedrich Engels. New York: International Publishers.

Marx, Karl, and Frederick Engels. 1970. *Manifesto of the Communist Party*. 3rd ed. Translated by Samuel Moore. Edited by Frederick Engels. Peking: Foreign Languages Press.

Maxwell, Angie, and Todd G. Shields. 2019. *The Long Southern Strategy: How Chasing White Voters in the South Changed American Politics*. New York: Oxford University Press.

Maxwell, Richard, and Toby Miller. 2016. "The Propaganda Machine behind the Controversy over Climate Science: Can You Spot the Lie in This Title?" *American Behavioral Scientist* 60, no. 3: 288–304.

———. 2020a. “Flat-Curvers vs. a Fat-Curve System: The Fight for the Future.” *Psychology Today*, April 7, 2020. https://www.psychologytoday.com/us/blog/greening-the-media/202004/flat-curvers-vs-fat-curve-system-the-fight-the-future.

———. 2020b. “After the Horror.” *Psychology Today*, April 30, 2020. https://www.psychologytoday.com/us/blog/greening-the-media/202004/after-the-horror.

———. 2020c. “No Justice, No Peace: On Pandemics, Race, and Environment.” *Psychology Today*, June 8, 2020. https://www.psychologytoday.com/us/blog/greening-the-media/202006/no-justice-no-peace-pandemics-race-and-environment.

Mayer, Jane. 2016. *Dark Money: The Hidden History of the Billionaires behind the Rise of the Radical Right*. New York: Doubleday.

Mazzucato, Mariana. 2015. *The Entrepreneurial State: Debunking Public vs. Private Sector Myths*. New York: Public Affairs.

———. 2020. “Capitalism after the Pandemic.” *Foreign Affairs*, November/December 2020. https://www.foreignaffairs.com/articles/united-states/2020-10-02/capitalism-after-covid-19-pandemic.

McDonnell, Patrick J., and Kate Linthicum. 2020. “As Vaccine Rollout Nears, Many Concerns Raised in Latin America, Hard Hit by COVID-19.” *Los Angeles Times*, December 20, 2020. https://www.latimes.com/world-nation/story/2020-12-20/vaccine-rollout-mexico-chile-latin-america-covid-19.

McPherson, Alan. 2016. *A Short History of U.S. Interventions in Latin America and the Caribbean*. Malden: Wiley-Blackwell.

Merton, Robert K. 1936. “The Unanticipated Consequences of Purposive Social Action.” *American Sociological Review* 1, no. 6: 894–904.

Meyerson, Harold, and Ernest Harburg. 1993. *Who Put the Rainbow in the Wizard of Oz: Yip Harburg, Lyricist*. Ann Arbor: University of Michigan Press.

Millán-Guerrero, Rebeca Oliva, Ramiro Caballero-Hoyos, and Joel Monárrez-Espino. 2020. “Poverty and Survival from COVID-19 in Mexico.” *Journal of Public Health*. https://doi.org/10.1093/pubmed/fdaa228.

Miller, J. D. B. 1984. "The Sovereign State and Its Future." *International Journal* 39, no. 2: 284–301.

Miller, Toby. 2008. *Makeover Nation: The United States of Reinvention*. Columbus: Ohio State University Press.

———. 2018. "Social Identities from Leicester to Latin London." *Social Identities: Journal for the Study of Race, Nation and Culture* 24, no. 1: 7–15.

Milton, John. 2005. *Paradise Lost*. Oxford: Oxford University Press.

Mirowski, Philip. 2011. *Science-Mart: Privatizing American Science*. Cambridge, Mass.: Harvard University Press.

Mirowski, Philip, and Dieter Plehwe, eds. 2009. *The Road from Mont Pèlerin: The Making of the Neoliberal Thought Collective*. Cambridge, Mass.: Harvard University Press.

Mitchell, Timothy. 2011. *Carbon Democracy: Political Power in the Age of Oil*. London: Verso.

Moderna. 2020. "Moderna's COVID-19 Vaccine Candidate Meets Its Primary Efficacy Endpoint in the First Interim Analysis of the Phase 3 COVE Study." November 16, 2020. https://investors.modernatx.com/news-releases/news-release-details/modernas-covid-19-vaccine-candidate-meets-its-primary-efficacy.

Moffatt, Barton, and Carl Elliott. 2007. "Ghost Marketing: Pharmaceutical Companies and Ghostwritten Journal Articles." *Perspectives in Biology and Medicine* 50, no. 1: 18–31.

Moffitt, Benjamin. 2016. *The Global Rise of Populism: Performance, Political Style, and Representation*. Stanford: Stanford University Press.

Morgenthau, Hans J., Kenneth W. Thompson, and David Clinton. 2005. *Politics among Nations*. Revised ed. New York: McGraw-Hill.

Mouffe, Chantal. 2018. *For a Left Populism*. London: Verso.

Mounk, Yascha. 2018. *The People vs. Democracy: Why Our Freedom Is in Danger and How to Save It*. Cambridge, Mass.: Harvard University Press.

Moynihan, Ray. 2004. "The Intangible Magic of Celebrity Marketing." *PLoS Medicine* 1, no. 2: 102–104.

Mudde, Cas, ed. 2017. *The Populist Radical Right: A Reader*. London: Routledge.

Mudde, Cas, and Cristóbal Rivera Kaltwasser. 2017. *Populism: A Very Short Introduction*. New York: Oxford University Press.

Muik, Alexander, Ann-Kathrin Wallisch, Bianca Sänger, Kena A. Swanson, Julia Mühl, Wei Chen, Hui Cai, Ritu Sarkar, Özlem Türeci, Philip R. Dormitzer, and Ugur Sahin. 2021. "Neutralization of SARS-CoV-2 Lineage B.1.1.7 Pseudovirus by BNT 162b2 Vaccine-Elicited Human Sera." *bioRxiv*. https://www.biorxiv.org/content/10.1101/2021.01.18.426984v1.

Mueller, Benjamin and Mitra Taj. (2020), 'La educación por televisión vive un auge por la pandemia del coronavirus', *New York Times*, 17 August. https://www.nytimes.com/es/2020/08/17/espanol/educacion-television.html.

Muller, Jan-Werner. 2016. *What Is Populism?* Philadelphia: University of Pennsylvania Press.

Nature. 2020a. "COVID Vaccines: The World's Medical Regulators Need Access to Open Data." 588:195.

———. 2020b. "Why *Nature* Supports Joe Biden for US President." 586:335.

———. 2021. "Why a Pioneering Plan to Distribute COVID Vaccines Equitably Must Succeed." 589:170.

Neidhöfer, Guido, Nora Lustig, and Mariano Tommasi. 2020. "Intergenerational Transmission of Lockdown Consequences: Prognosis of the Longer-Run Persistence of COVID-19 in Latin America." Commitment to Equity, Tulane University, Working Paper 99. http://repec.tulane.edu/RePEc/ceq/ceq99.pdf.

Nelson, Anne. 2019. *Shadow Network: Media, Money, and the Secret Hub of the Radical Right*. New York: Bloomsbury.

Nelson, Julie A. (2009). "Between a Rock and a Soft Place: Ecological and Feminist Economics in Policy Debates." *Ecological Economics* 69, no. 1: 1–8.

New England Journal of Medicine. 2020. "Dying in a Leadership Vacuum." 383:1479–1480.

Nguyet Erni, John. 1994. *Unstable Frontiers: Technomedicine and the Cultural Politics of "Curing" AIDS*. Minneapolis: University of Minnesota Press.

NIH. 2021. "Phase III Double-Blind, Placebo-Controlled Study of AZD7442 for Post-exposure Prophylaxis of COVID-19 Adults (STORM CHASER)." January 11, 2021. https://clinicaltrials.gov/ct2/show/NCT04625972.

North, Liisa L., and Timothy D. Clark, eds. 2018. *Dominant Elites in Latin America: From Neo-Liberalism to the "Pink Tide."* Cham: Palgrave Macmillan.

Nott, David. 2020. "The COVID-19 Response for Vulnerable People in Places Affected by Conflict and Humanitarian Crises." *Lancet* 395, no. 10236: P1532–P1533.

O'Donnell, Megan. 2020. "Preventing a 'Return to Normal': Addressing Violence against Women during COVID-19." Center for Global Development. November 24, 2020. https://www.cgdev.org/blog/preventing-return-normal-addressing-violence-against-women-during-covid-19.

OECD (Organisation for Economic Co-operation and Development). 2020. "Income Inequality." https://data.oecd.org/inequality/income-inequality.htm.

Office for National Statistics. 2020. "Crime in England and Wales: Year Ending March 2020." https://www.ons.gov.uk/peoplepopulationandcommunity/crimeandjustice/bulletins/crimeinenglandandwales/yearendingmarch2020#homicide.

———. 2021. "Personal and Economic Well-Being in Great Britain: January 2021." https://www.ons.gov.uk/peoplepopulationandcommunity/wellbeing/bulletins/personalandeconomicwellbeingintheuk/january2021.

Offner, Amy C. 2019. *Sorting Out the Mixed Economy: The Rise and Fall of Welfare and Developmental States in the Americas*. Princeton: Princeton University Press.

Olivarius, Kathryn. 2020. "The Dangerous History of Immunoprivilege." *New York Times*, April 12, 2020. https://www.nytimes.com/2020/04/12/opinion/coronavirus-immunity-passports.html.

Oltermann, Philip. 2020. "Scientist behind BioNTech/Pfizer Vaccine Says It Can End Pandemic." *Guardian*, November 12, 2020. https://www.theguardian.com/world/2020/nov/12/scientist-behind-biontech-pfizer-coronavirus-vaccine-says-it-can-end-pandemic.

One Health Initiative. n.d. https://onehealthinitiative.com.

OpenDemocracy. 2020. "Degrowth: New Roots for the Economy." https://www.opendemocracy.net/en/oureconomy/degrowth-new-roots-economy/.

Oquendo, Catalina. 2020. "El coronavirus no detiene la violencia en Colombia." *El País*, March 26, 2020. https://elpais.com/internacional/2020-03-26/el-coronavirus-no-detiene-la-violencia-en-colombia.html.

Orcutt, Miriam, Parth Patel, Rachel Burns, Lucinda Hiam, Rob Aldridge, Delan Devakumar, Bernadette Kumar, Paul Spiegel, and Ibrahim Abubakar. 2020. "Global Call to Action for Inclusion of Migrants and Refugees in the COVID-19 Response." *Lancet* 395, no. 10235: P1482–P1483.

Oreskes, Naomi, and Erik M. Conway. 2010. *Merchants of Doubt*. New York: Bloomsbury Press.

Osorio, Manuel. 1991. "Interview with Gabriel García Márquez." *Courier*. https://en.unesco.org/courier/octobre-1991/interview-gabriel-garcia-marquez.

Overy, Richard. 2020. "Why the Cruel Myth of the 'Blitz Spirit' Is No Model for How to Fight Coronavirus." *Guardian*, March 19, 2020. https://www.theguardian.com/commentisfree/2020/mar/19/myth-blitz-spirit-model-coronavirus.

Owen, Joseph. 2020. "States of Emergency, Metaphors of Virus, and COVID-19." *Verso*, March 31, 2020. https://www.versobooks.com/blogs/4636-states-of-emergency-metaphors-of-virus-and-covid-19.

OXFAM. 2016. "Unearthed: Land, Power, and Inequality in Latin America." https://www.oxfam.org/sites/www.oxfam.org/files/file_attachments/unearthed-executive-en-29nov-web.pdf.

———. 2020. "Campaigners Warn That 9 Out of 10 People in Poor Countries Are Set to Miss Out on COVID-19 Vaccine Next Year." December 9, 2020. https://www.oxfam.org/en/press-releases/campaigners-warn-9-out-10-people-poor-countries-are-set-miss-out-covid-19-vaccine.

PAHO (Pan American Health Organization). n.d. "Health Financing in the Americas." https://www.paho.org/salud-en-las-americas-2017/?p=178.

Palos, Mauricio. 2020. "'Planes Spray the City at Night': Covid-19 Conspiracy Theories in Mexico's Motor Town." *Guardian*, May 22, 2020. https://www.theguardian.com/global-development/2020/may/22/planes-spray-the-city-at-night-covid-19-conspiracy-theories-in-mexicos-motor-town.

Paltiel, A. David, Jason L. Schwartz, Amy Zheng, and Rochelle P. Walensky. 2021. "Clinical Outcomes of a COVID-19 Vaccine: Implementation over Efficacy." *Health Affairs* 40, no. 1: 42–52.

Panizza, Francisco, ed. 2005. *Populism and the Mirror of Democracy*. London: Verso.

Pardo, Daniel. 2019. "Paro nacional en Colombia: 3 factores inéditos que hicieron del 21 de noviembre un día histórico." *BBC Mundo*, November 22, 2019. https://www.bbc.com/mundo/noticias-america-latina-50520302.

Parkinson, Charles. 2020. "Three Women Murdered on First Day of Colombia's Coronavirus Lockdown." *Colombia Reports*, March 26, 2020. https://colombiareports.com/three-women-murdered-on-first-day-of-colombias-coronavirus-lockdown/.

Peace Alliance. 2015. "Key Statistics on the Challenges of Violence & Crime." https://peacealliance.org/wp-content/uploads/2013/05/statistics-on-violence-2015.pdf.

People and Corruption: Latin America and the Caribbean: Global Corruption Barometer. https://www.transparency.org/en/publications/global-corruption-barometer-people-and-corruption-latin-america-and-the-car

Pepys, Samuel. 2000. *The Diary of Samuel Pepys Volume VII: 1666*. Berkeley: University of California Press.

Perkins, Ellie and Edith Kuiper. (2005). "Introduction: Exploring Feminist Ecological Economics." *Feminist Economics* 11, no. 3: 107-10.

Peter, Zsombor. 2020. "Outbreak Sends Malaysia Scrambling to Test Migrant Workers." *VOA News*, May 10, 2020. https://www.voanews.com/covid-19-pandemic/singapores-coronavirus-outbreak-sends-malaysia-scrambling-test-migrant-workers.

Pfizer. 2020. "Pfizer and BioNTech Announce Vaccine Candidate against COVID-19 Achieved Success in First Interim Analysis from Phase 3 Study." November 9, 2020. https://www.pfizer.com/news/press-release/press-release-detail/pfizer-and-biontech-announce-vaccine-candidate-against.

Phillips, Tom. 2020. "Mexico Admits Covid Death Toll Much Higher Than Official Number." *Guardian*, October 26, 2020. https://www.theguardian.com/world/2020/oct/26/mexico-coronavirus-death-toll-much-higher-official-number.

Piketty, Thomas. 2014. *Capital in the Twenty-First Century*. Translated by Arthur Goldhammer. Cambridge, Mass.: Belknap Press of Harvard University Press.

———. 2018. "Brahmin Left vs Merchant Right: Rising Inequality & the Changing Structure of Political Conflict (Evidence from France, Britain and the US, 1948–2017)." WID.world Working Paper Series No. 2018/7. http://piketty.pse.ens.fr/files/Piketty2018.pdf.

Plato. 1972. *The Laws*. Translated by Trevor J. Saunders. Harmondsworth: Penguin.

Polack, Fernando P., Stephen J. Thomas, Nicholas Kitchin, Judith Absalon, Alejandra Gurtman, Stephen Lockhart, John L. Perez, Gonzalo Pérez Marc, Edson D. Moreira, Cristiano Zerbini, Ruth Bailey, Kena A. Swanson, Satrajit Roychoudhury, Kenneth Koury, Ping Li, Warren V. Kalina, David Cooper, Robert W. Frenck Jr., Laura L. Hammitt, Özlem Türeci, Haylene Nell, Axel Schaefer,

Serhat Ünal, Dina B. Tresnan, Susan Mather, Philip R. Dormitzer, Uğur Şahin, Kathrin U. Jansen, and William C. Grube. 2020. "Safety and Efficacy of the BNT162b2 mRNA Covid-19 Vaccine." *New England Journal of Medicine* 383:2603–2615.

Polanyi, Karl. 2001. *The Great Transformation: The Political and Economic Origins of Our Time*. Boston: Beacon Press.

Polese, Abel, Colin C. Williams, and Ioana A. Hordonic, eds. 2017. *The Informal Economy in Global Perspective: Varieties of Governance*. Cham: Springer.

Price, Carter C., and Kathryn A. Edwards. 2020. *Trends in Income from 1975 to 2018*. RAND Education and Labor. https://www.rand.org/pubs/working_papers/WRA516-1.html.

Pūras, Dainius, Judith Bueno de Mesquita, Luisa Cabal, Allan Maleche, and Benjamin Mason Meier. 2020. "The Right to Health Must Guide Responses to COVID-19." *Lancet* 395:1888–1890.

Quammen, David. 2012. *Spillover: Animal Infections and the Next Human Pandemic*. New York: W. W. Norton.

Quiggin, John. 2010. *Zombie Economics: How Dead Ideas Still Walk among Us*. Princeton: Princeton University Press.

Quintero Morales, Josefina. 2020. "Por la falta de ingresos, vendedores de Iztapalapa dicen 'no se guardarán.'" *La Jornada*, December 23, 2020. https://www.jornada.com.mx/notas/2020/12/23/capital/por-la-falta-de-ingresos-vendedores-de-iztapalapa-dicen-que-no-se-guardaran/.

Ramasubba Reddy, Indla, Jateen Ukrani, Visha Indla, and Varsha Ukrani. 2019. "Violence against Doctors: A Viral Epidemic?" *Indian Journal of Psychiatry* 61, suppl. 4: S782–S785.

Ramírez, Isabel Cristina, and Toby Miller. 2020. "Colombian Art 'under' Covid-19." In *Doing Arts Research in a Pandemic: A Crowd-Sourced Document Responding to the Challenges Arising from Covid-19*, compiled by Vida L. Midgelow, 19–20. London: Culture Capital Exchange.

Rangel, Clavel, Joe Parkin Daniels, and Tom Phillips. 2020. "'We're All on Death Row Now': Latin America's Prisons Reel from

Covid-19." *Guardian*, May 16, 2020. https://www.theguardian.com/world/2020/may/16/latin-america-prisons-covid-19-riots.

Rawls, John. 1971. *A Theory of Justice*. Cambridge, Mass.: Belknap Press of Harvard University Press.

Readfearn, Graham. 2015. "Was Climate Science Denialist Willie Soon Funded to Do Science or Was It Just PR Cash from the Fossil Fuel Industry?" *Desmog*, March 1, 2015. http://www.desmogblog.com/2015/03/01/was-climate-science-denialist-willie-soon-funded-do-science-or-was-it-just-pr-cash-fossil-fuel-industry.

Reich, Robert. 2020. "America Has No Real Public Health System." *Guardian*, March 15, 2020. https://www.theguardian.com/commentisfree/2020/mar/15/america-public-health-system-coronavirus-trump.

———. 2021. "Healthcare to the Electoral College: Seven Ways 2020 Left America Exposed." *Guardian*, January 3, 2021. https://www.theguardian.com/commentisfree/2021/jan/03/healthcare-electoral-college-covid-trump-seven-ways-2020-left-america-exposed.

Reinhart, Eric, and Daniel L. Chen. 2020. "Incarceration and Its Disseminations: COVID-19 Pandemic Lessons from Chicago's Cook County Jail." *Health Affairs* 39, no. 8: 1412–1418.

Renda, Andrea. 2018. *The Legal Framework to Address "Fake News": Possible Policy Actions at the EU Level*. European Parliament's Committee on the Internal Market and Consumer Protection. http://www.europarl.europa.eu/RegData/etudes/IDAN/2018/619013/IPOL_IDA(2018)619013_EN.pdf.

Rodrik, Dani. 2007. *One Economics, Many Recipes: Globalization, Institutions, and Economic Growth*. Princeton: Princeton University Press.

Roosevelt, Franklin Delano. 1933. "First Inaugural Address of Frankli D. Roosevelt." Yale Law School. https://avalon.law.yale.edu/20th_century/froos1.asp.

Roser-Renouf, Connie, Edward W. Maibach, Anthony Leiserowitz, and Xiaoquan Zhao. 2014. "The Genesis of Climate Change Activism: From Key Beliefs to Political Action." *Climatic Change* 125, no. 2: 163–178.

Ross, Andrew, ed. 1996. *Science Wars*. Durham: Duke University Press.

Roy, Arundhati. 2020. "The Pandemic Is a Portal." *Financial Times*, April 3, 2020. https://www.ft.com/content/10d8f5e8-74eb-11ea-95fe-fcd274e920ca.

Rupar, Aaron. 2020. "Jared Kushner's Ventilator Remarks Contradicted a Government Website. Hours Later, the Site Was Changed." *Vox*, April 3, 2020. https://www.vox.com/2020/4/3/21207140/jared-kushner-strategic-national-stockpile-ventilators.

Rusbridger, Alan. 2020. "Amid Our Fear, We're Rediscovering Utopian Hopes of a Connected World." *Guardian*, March 29, 2020. https://www.theguardian.com/commentisfree/2020/mar/29/coronavirus-fears-rediscover-utopian-hopes-connected-world.

Saez, Emmanuel. 2021. "Public Economics and Inequality: Uncovering Our Social Nature." American Economics Association Distinguished Lecture, January 2021. https://eml.berkeley.edu/~saez/ely-saez-slides_v3.pdf.

Said, Edward. 1999. "Hey, Mister, You Want Dirty Book?" *London Review of Books*, September 30, 1999. https://www.lrb.co.uk/the-paper/v21/n19/edward-said/hey-mister-you-want-dirty-book.

Saldarriaga H., Manuela. 2020. "La criminalización de la protesta social en Colombia es histórica." *Cerosetenta*, September 23, 2020. https://cerosetenta.uniandes.edu.co/la-criminalizacion-de-la-protesta-social-en-colombia-es-historica1/.

Sandilands, Catriona. 1999. *The Good-Natured Feminist: Ecofeminism and the Quest for Democracy*. Minneapolis: University of Minnesota Press.

Satomi, Erika, Polianna Mara Rodrigues de Souza, Beatriz de Costa Thomé, Claudio Reingenheim, Eduardo Werebe, Eduardo Juan Troster, Farah Christina de La Cruz Scarin, Hélio Arthur Bacha, Henrique Grunspun, Leonardo José Rolim Ferraz, Marco Aurelio Scarpinella Bueno, Mario Thadeu Leme de Barros Filho, and Pedro Custódio de Mello Borges. 2020. "Fair Allocation of Scarce Medical Resources during COVID-19 Pandemic: Ethical

Considerations." *Einstein* 18. https://www.scielo.br/scielo.php?script=sci_arttext&pid=S1679-45082020000100903.

Saunders, David. 1997. *Anti-lawyers: Religion and the Critics of Law and State*. London: Routledge.

Schleicher, Andreas. 2020. *The Impact of Covid-19 on Education: Insights from Education at a Glance 2020*. Organisation for Economic Co-operation and Development. http://www.oecd.org/education/the-impact-of-covid-19-on-education-insights-education-at-a-glance-2020.pdf.

Schreiber, Darren, Greg Fonzo, Alan N. Simmons, Christopher T. Dawes, TaruFlagan, James H. Fowler, and Martin P. Paulus. 2013. "Red Brain, Blue Brain: Evaluative Processes Differ in Democrats and Republicans." *PLoS ONE* 8, no. 2. http://journals.plos.org/plosone/article?id=10.1371/journal.pone.0052970.

Scientific American. 2020. "On November 3, Vote to End Attacks on Science." October 9, 2020. https://www.scientificamerican.com/article/on-november-3-vote-to-end-attacks-on-science/.

Sen, Amartya. 2009. *The Idea of Justice*. Cambridge, Mass.: Belknap Press of Harvard University Press.

Shaw, Timothy M., ed. n.d. *International Political Economy Series*. Cham: Palgrave Macmillan.

Shepherd, Ben, and Susan Stone. 2013. "Global Production Networks and Employment: A Developing Country Perspective." *OECD Trade Policy Papers* 154. http://dx.doi.org/10.1787/5k46j0rjq9s8-en.

Sheridan, Mary Beth, Niha Masih, and Regine Cabato. 2020. "As Coronavirus Fears Grow, Doctors and Nurses Face Abuse, Attacks." *Washington Post*, April 8, 2020. https://www.washingtonpost.com/world/the_americas/coronavirus-doctors-nurses-attack-mexico-ivory-coast/2020/04/08/545896a0-7835-11ea-a311-adb1344719a9_story.html.

Sieff, Kevin. 2020. "Mexican Factories Boost Production of Medical Supplies for U.S. Hospitals While Country Struggles with Its Own Coronavirus Outbreak." *Washington Post*, April 3, 2020. https://www.washingtonpost.com/world/the_americas/mexican

-medical-manufacturers-boost-production-for-us-hospitals-while-country-struggles-with-its-own-coronavirus-outbreak/2020/04/03/0e624fea-7517-11ea-ad9b-254ec99993bc_story.html.

Sin Embargo. 2020. "AMLO no ha logrado cambiar las causas que generan desigualdad en México, alerta Frente a la Probeza." September 1, 2020. https://www.sinembargo.mx/01-09-2020/3852531.

Singer, Merrill. 2020. "Deadly Companions: COVID-19 and Diabetes in Mexico." *Medical Anthropology* 39, no. 8: 660–665.

Singer, Merrill, Nicola Bulled, Bayla Ostrach, and Emily Mendenhall. 2017. "Syndemics and the Biosocial Conception of Health." *Lancet* 389:941–950.

Sismondo, Sergio. 2013. "Key Opinion Leaders and the Corruption of Medical Knowledge: What the Sunshine Act Won't Cast Light On." *Journal of Law, Medicine & Ethics* 41, no. 3: 635–643.

Sjoberg, Laura. 2013. *Gendering Global Conflict: Toward a Feminist Theory of War*. New York: Columbia University Press.

Slack, Jeremy, and Josiah Heyman. 2020. "Asylum and Mass Detention at the U.S.–Mexico Border during Covid-19." *Journal of Latin American Geography* 19, no. 3: 334–339.

Sliwa, Karen, and Magdi Yacoub. 2020. "Catalysing the Response to NCDI Poverty at a Time of COVID-19." *Lancet* 396:941–942.

Smith, Kimberly K. 2007. *African American Environmental Thought: Foundations*. Lawrence: University of Kansas Press.

Social Insurance and Allied Services: Report by Sir William Beveridge (Cmd. 6404). 1942. https://www.costsbarrister.co.uk/wp-content/uploads/2020/06/The-Beveridge-Report.pdf.

Soper, Kate. 1995. *What Is Nature? Culture, Politics and the Nonhuman*. Oxford: Blackwell.

Stein, Richard A., Oana Ometa, Sarah Pachtman Shetty, Adi Katz, Mircea Ionut Popitiu, and Robert Brotherton. 2021. "Conspiracy Theories in the Era of COVID-19: A Tale of Two Pandemics." *International Journal of Clinical Practice*. https://doi.org/10.1111/ijcp.13778.

StepChange. 2020. *Coronavirus and Personal Debt: A Financial Recovery Strategy for Households*. https://www.stepchange.org/Portals/0/assets/pdf/coronavirus-policy-briefing-stepchange.pdf.

Stevis-Grindneff, Matina. 2020. "The Rising Heroes of the Coronavirus Era? Nations' Top Scientists." *New York Times*, April 5, 2020. https://www.nytimes.com/2020/04/05/world/europe/scientists-coronavirus-heroes.html.

Stone, Diane. 2013. *Knowledge Actors and Transnational Governance: The Public-Private Policy Nexus in the Global Agora*. Basingstoke: Palgrave MacMillan.

Strange, Susan. 1997. *Casino Capitalism*. Manchester: Manchester University Press.

Sutton, Robbie M., and Karen M. Douglas. 2020. "Agreeing to Disagree: Reports of the Popularity of Covid-19 Conspiracy Theories Are Greatly Exaggerated." *Psychological Medicine*. https://doi.org/10.1017/S0033291720002780.

Synnott, Anthony. 2002. *The Body Social: Symbolism, Self and Society*. 2nd ed. London: Routledge.

Sze, Shirley, Daniel Pan, Clareece R. Nevill, Laura J. Gray, Christopher A. Martin, Joshua Nazareth, Jatinder S. Minhas, Pip Divall, Kamlesh Khunti, Keith R. Abrams, Laura B. Nellums, and Manish Pareek. 2020. "Ethnicity and Clinical Outcomes in COVID-19: A Systematic Review and Meta-analysis." *EClinicalMedicine* 29, no. 100630. https://www.thelancet.com/journals/eclinm/article/PIIS2589-5370(20)30374-6/fulltext.

Taggart, Paul. 2000. *Populism*. Buckingham: Open University Press.

Taylor, Louise H., Sophia M. Latham, and Mark E. J. Woolhouse. 2001. "Risk Factors for Human Disease Emergence." *Philosophical Transactions of the Royal Society B* 356, no. 1411: 983–989.

Taylor, Luke. 2020. "Covid-19 Misinformation Sparks Threats and Violence against Doctors in Latin America." *British Medical Journal* 370: m3088.

Tchekmedyian, Alene, and Richard Winton. 2020. "L.A. County Jail Inmates Trying to Infect Themselves with Coronavirus, Sheriff

Says." *Los Angeles Times*, May 11, 2020. https://www.latimes.com/california/story/2020-05-11/inmates-inside-la-county-jails-trying-to-intentional-infect-themselves-with-coronavirus-sheriff-says.

Thompson, Charis. 2006. "Back to Nature? Resurrecting Ecofeminism after Poststructuralist and Third-Wave Feminisms." *Isis* 97, no. 3: 505–512.

Tinson, Adam, and Amy Clair. 2020. *Better Housing Is Crucial for Our Health and the COVID-19 Recovery*. Health Foundation. https://www.health.org.uk/publications/long-reads/better-housing-is-crucial-for-our-health-and-the-covid-19-recovery.

Tollefson, Jeff. 2021. "COVID Curbed Carbon Emissions in 2020—but Not by Much." *Nature* 589:343.

Torrado, Santiago. 2020. "Sabemos que lo más duro está por venir." *El País*, April 26, 2020. https://elpais.com/sociedad/2020-04-26/sabemos-que-lo-mas-duro-esta-por-venir.html.

Treichler, Paula A. 1999. *How to Have Theory in an Epidemic: Cultural Chronicles of AIDS*. Durham: Duke University Press.

Trejos-Herrera, Ana M., Stefano Vinaccia, and Marly J. Bahamón. 2020. "Coronavirus in Colombia: Stigma and Quarantine." *Journal of Global Health* 10, no. 2: 1–5.

Tsai, Jack, and Michal Wilson. 2020. "COVID-19: A Potential Public Health Problem for Homeless Populations." *Lancet Public Health* 5, no. 4: E186–E187.

Turner, Patricia A. 1993. *I Heard It through the Grapevine: Rumor in African-American Culture*. Berkeley: University of California Press.

UNAIDS. 2020. "Uniting behind a People's Vaccine against COVID-19." May 14, 2020. https://www.unaids.org/en/resources/presscentre/featurestories/2020/may/20200514_covid19-vaccine-open-letter.

UNEP. 2020. *Emissions Gap Report*. https://www.unep.org/emissions-gap-report-2020.

UNEP and International Livestock Research Institute. 2020. *Preventing the Next Pandemic: Zoonotic Diseases and How to Break the*

Chain of Transmission. https://www.unenvironment.org/resources/report/preventing-future-zoonotic-disease-outbreaks-protecting-environment-animals-and.

UNICEF. 2020. "'The Future We Want': The Manifesto Written by Adolescents in Italy on the Post COVID-19 Future." https://www.unicef.org/eca/press-releases/future-we-want-manifesto-written-adolescents-italy-post-covid-19-future.

Urquieta-Salomón, José E., and Héctor J. Villarreal. 2016. "Evolution of Health Coverage in Mexico: Evidence of Progress and Challenges in the Mexican Health System." *Health Policy and Planning* 31, no. 1: 28–36.

Urrutia, Alonso. 2021. "El Presidente Andrés Manuel López Obrador da positivo a Covid." *La Jornada*, January 24, 2021. https://www.jornada.com.mx/notas/2021/01/24/politica/el-presidente-andres-manuel-lopez-obrador-da-positivo-a-covid/.

U.S. National Academies of Sciences, Engineering, and Medicine. 2020. "Discussion Draft of the Preliminary Framework for Equitable Allocation of COVID-19 Vaccine." https://www.nap.edu/catalog/25917/framework-for-equitable-allocation-of-covid-19-vaccine.

Van Lacker, Wim, and Zachary Parolin. 2020. "COVID-19, School Closures, and Child Poverty: A Social Crisis in the Making." *Lancet Public Health* 5, no. 5: E243–E244.

Varoufakis, Yanis. 2020. "A Chronicle of a Lost Decade Foretold." *Project Syndicate*, May 27, 2020. https://www.project-syndicate.org/commentary/bleak-preliminary-history-of-2020s-by-yanis-varoufakis-2020-05?barrier=accesspaylog.

Venegas, Juan Manuel. 2003. "¿Yo por qué?, insiste Fox; ¿qué no somos 100 millones de mexicanos?" *La Jornada*, August 2, 2003, Política 3.

Vickery, Jamie, and Lori M. Hunter. 2014. "Native Americans: Where in Environmental Justice Theory and Research?" Institute of Behavioral Science Population Program, University of Colorado Boulder Working Paper 4. http://www.colorado.edu/ibs/pubs/pop/pop2014-0004.pdf.

Virchow, Rudolf. 2006. "Report on the Typhus Epidemic in Upper Silesia." *American Journal of Public Health* 96, no. 12: 2102–2105.

Voysey, Merryn, Sue Ann Costa Clemens, Shabir A. Madhi, Lil Y. Weckx, Pedro M. Folegatti, Parvinder K. Aley, Brian Angus, Vicky L. Baillie, Shaun L. Barnabas, Qasim E. Bhorat, Sagida Bibi, Carmen Briner, Paola Cicconi, Andrea M. Collins, Rachel Colin-Jones, Clare L. Cutland, Thomas C. Darton, Keertan Dheda, Christopher J. A. Duncan, Katherine R. W. Emary, Katie J. Ewer, Lee Fairlie, Saul N. Faust, Shuo Feng, Daniela M. Ferreira, Adam Finn, Anna L. Goodman, Catherine M. Green, Christopher A. Green, Paul T. Heath, Catherine Hill, Helen Hill, Ian Hirsch, Susanne H. C. Hodgson, Alane Izu, Susan Jackson, Daniel Jenkin, Carina C. D. Joe, Simon Kerridge, Anthonet Koen, Gaurav Kwatra, Rajeka Lazarus, Alison M. Lawrie, Alice Lelliott, Vincenzo Libri, Patrick J. Lillie, Raburn Mallory, Ana V. A. Mendes, Eveline P. Milan, Angela M. Minassian, Alastair McGregor, Hazel Morrison, Yama F Mujadidi, Anusha Nana, Peter J. O'Reilly, Sherman D. Padayachee, Ana Pittella, Emma Plested, Katrina M. Pollock, Maheshi N. Ramasamy, Sarah Rhead, Alexandre V. Schwarzbold, Nisha Singh, Andrew Smith, Rinn Song, Matthew D. Snape, Eduardo Sprinz, Rebecc K. Sutherland, Richard Tarrant, Emma C. Thomson, M. Estée Török, Mark Toshner, David P. J. Turner, Johan Vekemans, Tonya L. Villafana, Marion E. E. Watson, Christopher J. Williams, Alexander D. Douglas, Adrian V. S. Hill, Teresa Lambe, Sarah C. Gilbert, Andrew J. Pollard. 2021. "Safety and Efficacy of the ChAdOx1 nCoV-19 Vaccine (AZD1222) against SARS-CoV-2: An Interim Analysis of Four Randomised Controlled Trials in Brazil, South Africa, and the UK." *Lancet* 397:P99–111.

Wabnitz, Katharina-Jaqueline, Sabine Gabrysch, Renzo Guinto, Andy Haines, Martin Herrmann, Courtney Howard, Teddie Potter, Susan L. Prescott, and Nicole Redver. 2020. "A Pledge for Planetary Health to Unite Health Professionals in the Anthropocene." *Lancet* 396:1471–1473.

Wade, Lizzie. 2020. "From Black Death to Fatal Flu, Past Pandemics Show Why People on the Margins Suffer Most." *Science*, May 14, 2020. https://www.sciencemag.org/news/2020/05/black-death-fatal-flu-past-pandemics-show-why-people-margins-suffer-most.

Wallace, Rob. 2016. *Big Farms Make Big Flu: Dispatches on Influenza, Agribusiness and the Nature of Science*. New York: Monthly Review Press.

Wallis, Victor, and Mingliang Zhuo. 2020. "Socialism, Capitalism, and the COVID-19 Epidemic: Interview with Victor Wallis." *International Critical Thought* 10, no. 2: 153–160.

Washington, Harriet A. 2020. "How Environmental Racism Is Fuelling the Coronavirus Pandemic." *Nature* 581:241.

Waters, Hannah. 2018. "How the U.S. Government Is Aggressively Censoring Climate Science." *Audobon*, Summer 2018. https://www.audubon.org/magazine/summer-2018/how-us-government-aggressively-censoring-climate.

Watts, Jonathan. 2020. "Bruno Latour: 'This Is a Global Catastrophe That Has Come from Within.'" *Guardian*, June 6, 2020. https://www.theguardian.com/world/2020/jun/06/bruno-latour-coronavirus-gaia-hypothesis-climate-crisis.

Webber, Jude. 2021. "Populist Amlo's Tight Grip on Mexico Finances Holds Back Covid Stimulus." *Financial Times*, January 12, 2021. https://www.ft.com/content/2bb141e2-4d0a-435f-9720-3f67b8077c28.

Webster, Paul Christopher. 2012a. "Health in Colombia: A System in Crisis." *Canadian Medical Association Journal* 184, no. 6: E289–E290.

———. 2012b. "Health in Colombia: Treating the Displaced." *Canadian Medical Association Journal* 184, no. 6: E291–E292.

Wenham, Clare, Julia Smith, and Rosemary Morgan. 2020. "COVID-19: The Gendered Impacts of the Outbreak." *Lancet* 395, no. 10227: P846–P848.

White, Roger. 2020. *Multidimensional Poverty in America: The Incidence and Intensity of Deprivation, 2008–2018*. Cham: Palgrave Macmillan.

Whitehead, Margaret, Ben Barr, and David Taylor-Robinson. 2020. "Covid-19: We Are Not 'All in It Together'—Less Privileged in

Society Are Suffering the Brunt of the Damage." *British Medical Journal*, May 22, 2020. https://blogs.bmj.com/bmj/2020/05/22/covid-19-we-are-not-all-in-it-together-less-privileged-in-society-are-suffering-the-brunt-of-the-damage/.

WHO. 2020a. "Disease Outbreak News: SARS-CoV-2 Variants." https://www.who.int/csr/don/31-december-2020-sars-cov2-variants/en/.

———. 2020b. "Making the Response to COVID-19 a Common Good: Solidarity Call to Action." https://www.who.int/docs/default-source/coronaviruse/solidarity-call-to-action/solidarity-call-to-action-01-june-2020.pdf?sfvrsn=a6c4b03d_4.

———. 2020c. "WHO Manifesto for a Healthy Recovery from COVID-19: Prescriptions and Actionables for a Healthy and Green Recovery." https://www.who.int/docs/default-source/climate-change/who-manifesto-for-a-healthy-and-green-post-covid-recovery.pdf?sfvrsn=f32ecfa7_8.

———. 2021. "COVID-19 Weekly Epidemiological Update." https://www.who.int/publications/m/item/weekly-epidemiological-update---12-january-2021.

WHO Ad Hoc Expert Group on the Next Steps for Covid-19 Vaccine Evaluation. 2021. "Placebo-Controlled Trials of Covid-19 Vaccines—Why We Still Need Them." *New England Journal of Medicine* 384. https://www.nejm.org/doi/10.1056/NEJMp2033538.

Wilkinson, Richard, and Kate Pickett. 2020. "Why Coronavirus Might Just Create a More Equal Society in Britain." *Guardian*, May 4, 2020. https://www.theguardian.com/commentisfree/2020/may/04/coronavirus-equal-society-britain-wellbeing-economic-growth.

Williams, Bruce A., and Michael Delli Carpini. 2011. *After Broadcast News: Media Regimes, Democracy, and the New Information Environment*. Cambridge: Cambridge University Press.

WINGX. 2021. "Business Aviation Weathers the Winter Blues." January 20, 2021. https://wingx-advance.com/business-aviation-weathers-the-winter-blues/.

World Bank. n.d.-a. "Hospital Beds (per 1,000 people)—Mexico." https://data.worldbank.org/indicator/SH.MED.BEDS.ZS?end=2018&locations=MX&start=1980.

———. n.d.-b. "Physicians (per 1,000 people)—Mexico." https://data.worldbank.org/indicator/SH.MED.PHYS.ZS?end=2018&locations=MX&start=1980.

World Economic Forum. 2021. *The Global Risks Report*. 16th ed. http://www3.weforum.org/docs/WEF_The_Global_Risks_Report_2021.pdf.

Wright, James. 2019. "Opinion: The Human Face of War." *Military Times*, June 27, 2019. https://www.militarytimes.com/opinion/2019/06/27/opinion-the-human-face-of-war/.

Yates, Luke. 2015. "Rethinking Prefiguration: Alternatives, Micropolitics and Goals in Social Movements." *Social Movement Studies: Journal of Social, Cultural and Political Protest* 14, no. 1: 1–21.

YouTube. 2010. "Churchill: 'This Is Not the End' (Nov. 1942)." May 15, 2010. https://www.youtube.com/watch?v=pdRH5wzCQQw&ab_channel=tototo981.

———. 2013. "Could You Patent the Sun?" January 29, 2013. https://www.youtube.com/watch?v=erHXKP386Nk.

———. 2021. "'A Year of Peace, a Year of Hope: Pope Francis Gives New Year's Blessing Despite Nerve Pain." January 1, 2021. https://www.youtube.com/watch?v=9RSBI3dUefo&ab_channel=EveningStandard.

Zavall, Lisa, Ezra M. Markowitz, and Elke U. Weber. 2015. "How Will I Be Remembered? Conserving the Environment for the Sake of One's Legacy." *Psychological Science* 26, no. 2: 231–236.

Zetterquist, Ola. 2011. "The Charter of Fundamental Rights and the European *Res Publica*." In *The EU Charter of Fundamental Rights: From Declaration to Binding Instrument*, edited by Giacomo Di Federico, 3–14. Dordrecht: Springer.

Index

About the Author

Toby Miller is the Stuart Hall Professor of Cultural Studies at the Universidad Autónoma Metropolitana-Cuajimalpa, Mexico City, and Sir Walter Murdoch Distinguished Collaborator at Murdoch University, Perth, Australia. The author and editor of over fifty books, his work has been translated into many languages. His most recent volumes are *Violence*, *The Persistence of Violence: Colombian Popular Culture*, and *How Green Is Your Cell Phone?*